Praise for Spectrum of Independence

"As a parent of three amazing children with autism spectrum disorder, I found this book very relatable, realistic, easy to follow, and an eye opener. Unlike other books on the same topic, it didn't leave me overwhelmed or confused! The authors write with a deep sense of empathy that truly shows their understanding of parents and kids. They masterfully explain how to guide children and organize their environment in a manner that sets them up for success and puts them on a path to becoming independent adults. The future seems a little less stressful and more achievable—for me, that is priceless."

—*Rachel O., Massapequa, New York*

"I love how straightforward and detailed this book is! It feels like the authors are having a conversation with you. The authors acknowledge that it will take work to teach your child daily life skills, but they also provide you with the exact steps needed to achieve your goals. This book has shifted my thinking and given me confidence. My daughter can now buckle her own seatbelt—a major accomplishment for us!"

—*Kathryn S., Wantagh, New York*

"I have worked with learners of all ages. What makes this book so special is its heart. It goes beyond just teaching basic tasks. It is a roadmap for creating lifelong learning experiences rooted in empathy, empowerment, and support. Whether you are just starting your journey or are looking for a fresh approach, this book needs to be part of your toolbox for helping your child build a joyful and independent life."

—*Tara Karen, MSEd, BCBA, LBA, Director of Service Provision, Achieve Beyond Pediatric Therapy and Autism Services*

"The authors provide calm, pragmatic advice and give you a framework for proactively building your child's skills. I will recommend this book to all of the parents I work with."

—*Sarah Hansen, PhD, Associate Professor of Special Education, Georgia State University*

"I've often tried to teach my son an everyday routine and given up because I didn't have the tools needed to succeed. This book has been tremendously useful to break down skills that may seem like second nature to typically developing children. So many of the scenarios made me stop and say, 'This is exactly what I needed!' I feel like I can breathe a little easier now. Sometimes it feels as though all the schooling, home therapy, and other therapy takes up a lot of our life, and we forget to stop and enjoy our child. That has changed after reading this book—it has lifted my spirits and given me hope."
—*Erica K., Levittown, New York*

"This is a great resource for any parent, like myself, who sees a future for their neurodiverse child that includes independent living, but isn't quite sure how to navigate the steps needed to prepare, support, and empower their child to thrive. I particularly enjoy the vignettes. They have the right level of detail and are varied enough to encompass different families' experiences. The suggested activities are well thought out and well presented."
—*Bryan S., Massapequa Park, New York*

"A 'must read' for any parent of a neurodiverse child. *Spectrum of Independence* is a compassionate, practical guide filled with insights and steps to help children take ownership of their daily routines. Reading this book, it feels like the authors are speaking directly to you, offering genuine support and encouragement. This book is a go-to for families looking to create structure and foster self-reliance while celebrating every step forward."
—*Jing Zhou, MS, BCBA, Founder, Alpine Academy, Oviedo, Florida*

Spectrum of Independence

Spectrum of Independence

HOW TO TEACH YOUR NEURODIVERSE CHILD DAILY LIFE SKILLS

Kristin Lombardi, MA
Christine Drew, PhD

Foreword by Peter Gerhardt, EdD

THE GUILFORD PRESS
New York   London

Copyright © 2025 The Guilford Press
A Division of Guilford Publications, Inc.
www.guilford.com

All rights reserved

The information in this volume is not intended as a substitute for consultation with health care professionals. Each individual's health concerns should be evaluated by a qualified professional.

Purchasers of this book have permission to copy select materials, where indicated by footnotes, for personal use or use with clients. These materials may be copied from the book or accessed directly from the publisher's website, but may not be stored on or distributed from intranet sites, internet sites, or file-sharing sites, or made available for resale. No other part of this book may be reproduced, translated, stored in a retrieval system, or transmitted, in any form or by any means, electronic, mechanical, photocopying, microfilming, recording, or otherwise, without written permission from the publisher.

Printed in the United States of America

This book is printed on acid-free paper.

Last digit is print number: 9 8 7 6 5 4 3 2 1

Library of Congress Cataloging-in-Publication Data is available from the publisher.

ISBN 978-1-4625-5491-1 (paperback) — ISBN 978-1-4625-5717-2 (hardcover)

*To all of the families that we have had the honor
of working with and learning from*

Contents

Authors' Note — ix

Foreword — xi

Acknowledgments — xv

Introduction — 1

PART I
Creating a New Future

1 "Why Aim for Independent Living?": — 9
   Your Child's Reality Now and in the Future

2 "How Am I Supposed to Do This?": — 23
   Leveraging the Power of Task Analysis

PART II
Assessment

3 "Is My Child Ready for This?": — 35
   Evaluating Your Child's Readiness

4 "Are You Ready for This?": — 61
   Evaluating Your Own Readiness

PART III
The Basics of Learning

5 "What Do I Need to Know before I Start?":   85
Understanding Behavior

6 "How Am I Going to Teach?":   104
Empowering versus Enabling

PART IV
Let's Do This!

7 "How Do I Start?":   129
How to Create a Task Analysis

8 "How Do I Get Myself Out of the Routine?":   164
Fading Prompts to Build Independence

PART V
Maximizing Independence

9 "When Do I Modify the Goal?":   179
Accommodating the Child versus Modifying the Goal

Epilogue. "How Do I Keep Moving Forward?":   197
Expanding Your Child's Independence

Glossary   199

References   203

Index   205

About the Authors   214

Purchasers of this book can download and print enlarged versions
of select materials at *www.guilford.com/lombardi-forms* for
personal use or use with clients (see copyright page for details).

Authors' Note

We have used the customary clinical terms from the fields of education and behavior intervention. Increased familiarity with these terms can help facilitate communication between you and your child's providers. This book includes stories to help illustrate the spectrum of neurodiversity and our approach to teaching life skills. These stories are either fictional, composite, or thoroughly disguised to protect individuals' privacy.

Foreword

Over my four-decade career, personal independence for individuals with an *intellectual or developmental disability (IDD)* has received significant attention as a concept but less attention as an actual life skill. Part of the problem is that we, in our roles as parents, educators, behavior analysts, and the like, spend too much time discussing deficits and not enough time discussing the potential for independence. By way of example, the number of skills that I don't have in my repertoire far exceeds the number of skills I do have in my repertoire. Yet rarely, if ever, does anyone say, "Peter is a smart guy, but he can't (1) hammer a nail in straight, (2) speak Vietnamese, (3) dance in any way that looks natural, (4) keep bees, or (5) dunk a basketball." The same, unfortunately, cannot be said for individuals with an IDD. That may be even more true when discussing independence.

Independence can be a very scary concept. This is not because independence isn't a desirable goal—I think we would all agree it is. Independence can be scary because an unfortunate side effect of independence is an increased exposure to risk. It is one thing to be independent in dressing (a very important skill), but dressing does not carry the same level of risk as crossing the street, using the stove, adjusting the water temperature before taking a shower, or riding a bicycle around the block.

Historically, the way such risk was minimized, if not eliminated entirely, was not to let adolescents and adults with an IDD engage in any sort of generalized independence. Instead, individuals were supervised throughout the day, and these supervisors, whether parents or nonparent professionals, were primarily there to make sure nothing bad happened. They controlled for the risk. Sadly, this continual supervision resulted in a "culture of dependence" where the independence displayed by the IDD adult was, at best, discouraged or, at worst, punished.

Thankfully, that is changing, and personal independence is increasingly targeted for acquisition across diverse environments, including the community. With the publication of Kristin Lombardi and Christine Drew's *Spectrum of Independence: How to Teach Your Neurodiverse Child Daily Life Skills*, there is no longer any good reason not to prioritize this critically important adolescent and adult skill. Framing personal independence in the context of taking ownership of the process is one of the most critical and useful aspects of this book. Ownership recognizes that skills that are personally valued by an individual (that is, ones they like to do or that provide them with some desired payoff) are often acquired quickly and maintained in their repertoire as they are regularly practiced. This is the difference between watching preferred videos on an iPad versus doing a math worksheet on an iPad. In most cases, watching preferred videos would fall into the highly valued category as opposed to the math worksheet, which likely would not.

Most people, by the way, value ownership of their daily living routines. It is something of a control function, I think. People do things the way they do them because they want to do them that way, and they have been reinforced over time for doing them the way they do. What matters is that each routine results in the desired, acceptable outcome. While there is currently little need to actually sort laundry before washing, I sort laundry. But I sort laundry by function, not color. Pants go in one load. Button-down shirts in another. T-shirts and underwear in yet another, while socks make up the final load. Don't mess with my routine, and I will always have clean clothes, and that is the only reason to do laundry in the first place. Ownership and independence go hand in hand.

So, you should consider yourself very lucky to have a copy of this gem of a book either in your hand or on your screen. I do not say that lightly. This book is a gem. Do yourself a favor. Actually read this book. Don't just flip through it or leave it in a pile on your desk for three months before putting it on a shelf with other unread books. Read it, take notes, use Post-its to highlight important sections, and then use what you have read in your home, classroom, or clinic. Remember, this is a process, and no one becomes independent in their daily living routines overnight.

From early on in my career, I was taught that independence was more important than perfection. It is true. On any given day, I demonstrate probably 85% accuracy across all tasks. At the same time, I am close to 100% independent across all tasks in all environments. That distribution has served me well. At the end of the day, everyone can become more independent as long as you work with them in that process. At the risk of repeating myself, *read this book!*

PETER GERHARDT, EdD
The EPIC Programs, Paramus, New Jersey
Endicott College, Beverly, Massachusetts

Acknowledgments

First, we would like to thank all of the families, clients, and students we have had the pleasure of working with and learning from over the past 20 years.

We especially want to thank all our parent readers who contributed their time, personal experience, and insights throughout the creation of this book. Without your input and feedback, this would be a very different (and probably less helpful) book.

This book would not have come to be, if it were not for the insightful and keen guidance of Marisa Solis, who patiently led us through the process of creating both the proposal and manuscript.

We are extremely grateful for Kitty Moore's enthusiasm and support. Her belief in our idea, and her trust in us as authors, were invaluable. We want to thank our team at The Guilford Press—Lucy Baker, Rebecca Bender, Anna Brackett, and Paul Gordon—for their excitement and expertise in carrying the book through its final stages of creation.

Huge thanks to Sarah Hansen, Tara Karen, and Jing Zhou, who took time out of their busy days to proof our manuscript and offer their professional opinions.

A special thanks to Chris Gorges and Jameson Tibbs—for their brilliant minds, attention to detail, and steadfast guidance.

Last but not least, we thank our friends, families, and partners for listening to us celebrate, lament, and talk about this book for the last two years. We appreciate your ears, patience, and insights!

Introduction

The majority of American parents don't have to think twice about their child's readiness to go to college, enter the workforce, or move out of the family home after high school. Unfortunately, this luxury is not afforded to all parents, especially those of neurodiverse children. Although the term neurodiverse was initially coined in reference to people on the autism spectrum, its usage has since become broader, including all people whose brains work differently than a "neurotypical" brain. Today, the term neurodiverse can be used to describe people with autism spectrum disorder, intellectual disability, developmental disabilities, ADHD, genetic disorders such as Down syndrome, and many more. These neurodiverse individuals may have great strengths in certain areas and achieve success. However, these individuals also commonly experience varying degrees of impairments and barriers across physical, cognitive, communication, social, and behavioral domains, which can make it difficult for them to get through the day without a lot of support.

As a parent of a neurodiverse child, you already face additional—and mostly unseen by others—logistical responsibilities. These include providing your child an exceptionally high level of care and supervision, coordinating additional care, dealing with the medical system, navigating special education, and handling the endless frustrations of managing federal and state benefits. This is on top of your job, community commitments, and personal and family relationships. Phew! Your resources are thin, and your energy is drained. You're stressed and worried about your child's current progress. This is not at all what you had imagined for them before learning about their developmental and learning differences. You likely had big plans for your child like graduating high school, attending college, securing an amazing job, getting married, and eventually living on their own—all while surrounded by a great group of friends. And so, you might be losing hope that your child will ever accomplish these things. Whether your child is 8 or 18, you're looking into their future and are uncertain about what it holds. It's a scary place to be.

As you read in the foreword, Dr. Peter Gerhardt discusses how, with the best of intentions, we spent decades overhelping people with developmental disabilities, which created a culture of dependence. We want to be part of the movement trying to course correct that mentality. And we want you to join us. We are asking you to reimagine what your child's future could look like. They may not earn a bachelor's degree, but that doesn't mean that their education needs to end when they turn 21 and transition out of public school services. What if they could attend a 4-year inclusive higher education college program? They may not hold an executive position in a big company, but that doesn't mean they can't be gainfully employed. What if they could get a paid job that they love, work with people that respect them, and feel fulfilled at the end of each day? They may not be able to live completely independently, but that doesn't mean that they need to spend the rest of their life living with you. What if they could live on their own with a roommate, frequent check-ins, or a part-time assistant? Independence looks different for everyone.

Reimagining your child's future is likely an exciting yet daunting process that will evolve over time. We see you. In fact, we created this book for you. *Spectrum of Independence: How to Teach Your Neurodiverse Child Daily Life Skills* is a result of a combined 37 years working with neurodiverse children and their parents. The title pays tribute to the fact that independence exists on a spectrum; it is not black and white. We all fall somewhere along this spectrum.

As board certified behavior analysts (BCBAs), we've witnessed firsthand the achievement that is possible when children with disabilities are taught in a way that makes sense to them. That's what we hope this book will do for you—teach you how to analyze, approach, and break down daily living activities for your child so that they can successfully learn to complete the tasks on their own. The "breaking down" of tasks—such as brushing teeth and making a sandwich—will happen to such a minute degree that skill development becomes manageable and doable for your child. In other words, not just baby steps, but microsteps.

This process, called *task analysis,* is an evidence-based practice. This means that this book's entire approach to teaching your child independent living skills is rooted in science. This approach has been effective for the many families we've worked with, and it can be for you too. We have broken this book into five parts, with guiding questions in each chapter. And here is the best part—just like developmental disabilities fall across a wide spectrum, so can one's success with this book. It is not so much a matter of if your child can "master" the skills in this book, but can they get to a place that is better (more independent) then where they started.

You can think of Part I of this book as addressing the "why": why increasing independence matters, along with a brief overview of the science of behavior. In Part II, we'll talk about the "who": your child and you. You'll assess your child's readiness and then your own readiness to complete the activities in this book. In Part III, you'll get information on the "what": behavior and prompting, the key factors in this program. In Part IV, you will get the "how": you'll learn to make a task analysis for your child and how to use it, how to gradually remove yourself from the routine, and how to make the routine accessible for your child. Finally, in Part V, we finish with the "when": knowing when to accommodate your child versus modifying the task.

With this book, you will learn how to do the following:

- Increase your child's responsibility for their daily living routines.
- Minimize or eliminate yourself from your child's self-care routines.
- Apply these techniques across several domains, including self-care, home living, and social interactions.
- Ease communication between your family and the professionals helping your child through shared behavioral vocabulary.

In addition, you will likely have boosted your child's self-confidence and self-efficacy in the process!

And as an added bonus, as your child becomes more independent, you will regain leisure time and newfound mental energy for yourself. Many of you are probably spread so thin that you have been neglecting time with other family members, hobbies, and self-care. As you regain that time, you may find you can give attention to people and activities that have long been overlooked.

Work Smarter, Not Harder

But here's the ticket, if you want a future characterized by more independence for your child and more freedom for yourself, *you will need to do things differently*. Think of it as working *smarter* toward your child's future, rather than *harder*. Though we will be frank, there will undoubtedly be some hard work along the way. We wrote this book to show you the main tools we have been using for years, and how to adapt them for yourself and your child. We understand your struggle and want you to know that life can likely get easier—for you and your child—if you commit to the strategies in this book.

Independent living skills are critical to your child's success now and as they grow. The tough part, though, is that your life might get a bit harder before it gets easier. This is the reality of anything we learn in life, from how to ride a bike to how to navigate a new area the first time. We will teach you how to create and use a task analysis, and you will teach your child how to execute that task analysis as independently as possible. Eventually, this can lead to your child learning to function more independently throughout the day.

This will require time, energy, and a commitment from you. We understand your reserves in this area are already low. But we are asking you to find a way to recharge your battery so that you can join us in learning a method that will give you less stress and more peace of mind in the near future, knowing that your child can likely do a lot more for themselves than they currently are.

Here's what we will ask of you in this book:

- To look into your child's future and at the potential that lies there
- To look in detail at what your child does daily
- To address any barriers in your home environment
- To be willing to change your interactions with your child
- To increase your expectations for your child
- To break down activities into microsteps using task analysis
- To track your child's progress

We know that your attention to this book and the activities in it will increase your to-do list in the short term, but our hope is that it will decrease your stress and worries in the long term. Your consistency and follow-through are imperative to your child's success. Your child needs you on their team, and actively moving them forward toward independent living, in order for this to work. Their age doesn't matter. What matters is your commitment to a new and different kind of work now, so that there's less work for you and more independence for your child in the future. The time you put in now will save you time and frustration in the future. Reading this book and completing the activities in it are an investment in yourself and your child.

We're asking you to be efficient and to give yourself the space needed to focus on your work with your child. New things can be scary, and you may experience resistance from your own internal thoughts, from therapists that work with your child, and even from family members that barely know your child. You will probably even experience resistance directly from your child, who may understandably be frustrated that you have stopped doing so much for them and are now expecting them to do things for themselves! We urge you to look past this resistance, though, and work through the book with an open mind. This will give you the best chance to see for yourself what your child is truly capable of accomplishing.

We hope the vignettes provided throughout the book offer you reassurance that your daily struggles are felt by others, allow you to see places in your child's life where dependence can become independence, and create a sense of optimism for what your and your child's future may hold.

Part I

Creating a New Future

1

"Why Aim for Independent Living?"

YOUR CHILD'S REALITY NOW AND IN THE FUTURE

"Jamie, time to wake up," Taylor whispers to her son for the third time this morning. He grumbles and rolls over. She picks him up and places him on his feet, knowing if he's not up on his own by now, she must intervene. He rubs his eyes and sits on the floor. Taylor says, "Time to potty," but Jamie stays on the floor until his mother lifts him to standing again. She points toward the bathroom and says firmly, "Go potty." Jamie walks to the bathroom still rubbing his eyes and yawning. He uses the bathroom and returns to his bedroom. Taylor cocks her head to one side and taps his shoulder to get his attention. "I didn't hear the flush. Go flush the toilet and wash your hands." Jamie goes back and flushes the toilet before returning. She sends him back again to wash his hands. He does as he's told, then returns with wet hands that don't smell like soap, and water down the front of his pajamas. Taylor sighs and walks him back into the bathroom, points at the soap, and says, "Use soap," before turning on the faucet. She then takes Jamie's hands, places one under the pump and one on top and presses down until soap comes out. Then she rubs Jamie's hands together under the faucet. Once he's done and she follows him back to his room, she points to the outfit that she has laid out on the bed. She says in a tired voice, though the day has only just begun, "Time to get dressed. It's picture day today."

Sound familiar? The morning routine can be one of the most demanding parts of the day. And the rush to get everyone to school and work on time adds pressure none of us need. The reality is, your days are long. Hectic. Sometimes they feel monotonous. You may feel like a broken record having to give the same directions and reminders day in and day out to your child with a developmental or intellectual disability. You manage to get your child off to school, but your duties don't end there. Let's meet Mark, whose 12-year-old son, Andy, has autism.

The phone rings as Mark types up a proposal at work. It's Andy's speech therapist with an update from his latest assessment. She confirms what Mark feared—Andy's social pragmatic language skills are still significantly delayed for his age, and he is struggling to engage with his peers during academic and social time. As Mark's heart sinks, the therapist recommends they look into a social skills group at the local university. She reminds Mark that helping Andy improve his communication skills will probably decrease the number of arguments he is having in class. This is a big goal for his individualized education program (IEP) team. Mark jots down the name of the professor in charge of the groups, knowing this means more research for him to do and yet another appointment on both Andy's and Mark's already overcrowded calendars.

Mark is still processing this news when his cellphone buzzes five minutes later. It's Andy's teacher, telling Mark that Andy had a difficult morning and a conflict with his group during math. Andy has calmed down now but refuses to rejoin class to finish the day's lessons. Mark glances wistfully at his coworker Jane, who is arranging a new set of framed photos of her two neurotypical children on her desk. The oldest just left home for college, and the youngest, the same age as Andy, made it to the state competition for speech and debate. "I'll be there in 20 minutes," Mark tells the teacher reluctantly.

Scheduling can be a nightmare. And if you have other children, you are likely over your limit managing pickups, drop-offs, dentist appointments, sports practices, games, competitions, lessons, family events, and therapy sessions. It can be overwhelming and nonstop. Your responsibilities may not end even after your child graduates from high school or a transition program. For many families of children with disabilities, these responsibilities can be lifelong. Let's meet Mariela and her 19-year-old daughter Janie, who has a rare genetic disorder and an intellectual disability.

"Let's do the checklist," Mariela tells her daughter. "Wallet, phone, keys, and lanyard," replies Janie. "That's right, and don't forget to remind the manager that you need to leave at 2." "Mommmm, I know, it's in my calendar app. Geez." Mariela smiles at her daughter's slightly sarcastic response and accompanying eye roll. Janie knows the drill. She's been working at the local grocery store in the bakery for almost three months now and has the routine down pat.

When Mariela goes to pick Janie up a few hours later for her appointment, she's surprised to see Janie in tears. Janie tells her that her boss had forgotten to get coverage for the second half of her shift, so when she reminded him about her appointment, he had asked if she could stay later. Mariela froze. Two of Janie's big triggers are schedule changes and missing appointments. Janie said that it took her "a long time" to calm down and that she was "stuck" on missing her appointment. She said, "Mom, I just kept telling him that I have to go. I have to go. But he didn't listen to me."

On the drive to the appointment, Mariela panicked. She knew she was catastrophizing, but all her worries about Janie's future, along with a long list of what-ifs, came flooding into her mind. What if Janie was fired? This was the first job she'd been able to keep. She loved her coworkers, and the schedule worked great with other family obligations. Would the store have eventually called the police if she hadn't calmed down? Should Mariela have talked to the manager instead of having Janie do it herself? She wanted Janie to be independent, but that seemed so far away still.

For all parents, the worries don't end when their child graduates from high school and gets a job. But for parents of children with disabilities, those worries are often bigger and more complex, as is their role in their child's life. Many times, parents and family members continue to have an outsized presence in their young adult and adult children's lives. This role may include advocacy, transportation, guardianship, decision making, and other types of support.

Indeed, you have a lot on your plate. You're juggling more than most people, and you may be worried you'll be inundated with the same obligations the rest of your life. We have seen firsthand how these worries can wreak havoc on families in the short and long term.

Your worries are not unfounded. The research paints a dim picture of what a child with an intellectual or developmental disability has to look forward to as an adult. In our work, we see clearly how independent living skills promote healthy lifestyles and thriving families. On the flip side, we also witness what happens when families neglect to teach their child with intellectual or developmental disabilities independent living skills while they are still young. When these children turn into young adults who still lack these skills, the effects can be devastating. This is true for all of us, but it is particularly impactful for children with intellectual or developmental disabilities and their families. We share this information with you not to discourage you, but to provide an honest depiction of what your child's future could hold if the proper supports are not put in place now. Let's look at what the data tell us, so that you can understand the full context in which you are operating.

What the Research Tells Us

In general, people with *autism spectrum disorder* (ASD) and an *intellectual disability* (ID) are doing particularly poorly when they exit high school or the K–12 system. Longitudinal data on adults with ASD find that about half (49.3%) have poor outcomes related to social involvement (friends and relationships), competitive employment, and independent living (Mason et al., 2021). One study found that adaptive skills are an important factor that influences living situation, employment, education, and physical health outcomes (Forbes et al., 2023). So, what this tells us is that teaching children adaptive skills using task analysis may have a significant impact on their future success.

In the next sections we present real-world scenarios of what families face every day while helping their children navigate the world of independent living. We present these illustrative stories alongside current research detailing long-term outcomes for people with ID across domains.

Lack of Services and Service Providers after Graduation

> Rosa crossed her fingers as she called the seventh therapist on her list. Her son Raul, a 19-year-old with autism and an intellectual disability, was struggling with inappropriate behavior in his dayhab and was on the verge of being removed from the program. Due to the seriousness of the behavior, his social worker suggested finding a behavior analyst (this may refer to a Board Certified Behavior Analyst [BCBA] or licensed behavior analyst [LBA]) to take on Raul's case. Rosa had contacted so many providers, she basically had a script memorized. Yes, they had insurance. No, they could not afford private pay. No, he was not in school, so there was no school

district to foot the bill either. Yes, he needed support in the community. No, a clinical setting would not work for him. Thus far everyone she spoke to was either booked, private pay only, or only worked with young children. She knew it wouldn't be easy to find a provider, but she didn't think it would be this tough.

The dayhab program was fine, but essentially amounted to day care for adults. Raul didn't really like going there. It was only for two days a week, but Rosa needed those two days so she could work her freelance job and take care of things around the house. It was up to Rosa to create Raul's programming for the rest of the week. They went to the movies on Mondays, shopped together on Tuesdays, and had Special Olympics on Thursdays. This wasn't enough. Raul needed more, and she was worried that his behavior would mean she'd be looking for another dayhab program soon too. Rosa sighed and dialed again.

Many people with disabilities and their families feel that leaving the K–12 system is like falling off a cliff in terms of services, community, and opportunities. There are also precious few resources at the local, state, and federal level for adults with ID and ASD, which becomes particularly stressful if a family cannot afford to pay for private services. The system is "ill-prepared and underfunded" and presents a "looming crisis of unprecedented magnitude for adults with autism and their families" (Gerhardt & Lainer, 2011).

Many practitioners only work with younger populations. Therapists are also not transition specialists and may not be familiar with the resources available to young people with disabilities after they graduate. Insurance may be unwilling to cover services that had been previously provided by school districts or transition programs. These issues may seem far away, but most parents report that the old adage of "the days are long, but the years are short" really holds true and that their children arrive at adulthood and transition more quickly than they realize. This is our inspiration for talking about these issues early and often with parents of children, even before adolescence.

Postsecondary Education

Jordan had always been interested in cars, so his mother, Maya, started to research mechanic and car tech programs in their area. Unfortunately, those programs required a regular diploma from an accredited high school or a GED for their applications, and Jordan had only received a certificate of completion for an alternate diploma. The high school that Jordan attended had a vocational feeder program for mechanics, but Jordan wasn't eligible to participate because he was in the Life Skills program and the mechanics teacher wasn't willing to work with the Life Skills teacher or Maya.

Maya was incredibly frustrated with the high school and with Jordan's options for education after graduation. He attended school until he was 21, and then Maya felt like they'd been dumped by the school system and his transition program with no plan in place. He'd been added to waiting lists for day programs and Maya was left to organize everything for his schedule and his daily life. She began looking at the inclusive higher education program at the local university, but soon realized that the price tag was far too much for them. She wasn't sure what to do now.

The *Individuals with Disabilities Education Act*, or IDEA, does not apply to colleges, universities, or postsecondary education of any kind. So, the right to access education after high school is not guaranteed. While students are still covered by *Section 504 of the Rehabilitation Act of 1973* after high school, those protections are very limited when compared with IDEA. Section 504 forbids discrimination within any organization that accepts federal funding, but only allows for accommodations that don't create an "undue burden" or "fundamentally alter" an activity. While there are increasing opportunities for postsecondary education through inclusive higher education programs, there are currently only about 300 of these programs nationwide, with very limited capacity (*https://thinkcollege.net*). Some programs receive 10 times more applications than the number of students they can admit. Many of these programs also require students to attain minimum levels of proficiency in reading and math, the ability to be left unsupervised for several hours or even 24 hours at a time, and mastery of basic safety behaviors like being safe on a college campus or crossing streets. Many young people with ASD and ID simply do not qualify for inclusive higher education programs, and even if they do, it does not guarantee acceptance into a program due to the limited number of spots available.

Another factor is the cost. There are now more options for funding for postsecondary education through state-level workforce or vocational rehabilitation programming. However, these concessions are hard won by parents advocating their state programs and lobbying for new laws allowing for this funding to be used. These programs also may not qualify students for loans or grants through *Free Application for Federal Student Aid*, or FAFSA, as it's commonly known. The steep cost is often more than families can afford, particularly since most families did not know these programs existed when their children were young, so they missed out on opportunities to save.

There are also vocational training programs for jobs such as cosmetology, welding, or health care roles such as nursing aides, but these require students to have obtained a high school diploma, complete a rigorous certification process, take written and practical exams, and participate in internships. The coursework and exams needed to obtain these certifications are usually fairly rigid and therefore do not lend themselves to accommodations. If students are accepted, the challenges continue; students must keep up with the pace of coursework, and while some instructors may be willing to provide supports, these would be on an individual basis and are not guaranteed. These programs also come with a hefty price tag that must be paid up front or through loans. Either way, these programs may be out of reach for many families.

Social Connections or Friend Networks

Dori clenched her phone in her hand. Her friend Emily hadn't texted her back. Dori texted again, for the 30th time. She'd also called, sent Instagram messages, and tried to FaceTime Emily. Dori has Down syndrome, and seeing and talking with her friends was important to her, especially since she'd left her transition program at the high school and her social connections had dwindled. She knew she shouldn't text and call too much, but she just couldn't seem to help herself. When her mom knocked on her door and came to sit on her bed, she knew she was in trouble. Molly, Dori's mom, said she wasn't "in trouble" but let her know that Emily's mom had reached out to her. Molly told her that Emily didn't want to talk to her and so she had blocked her number for a while. Molly said that Dori needed to respect that boundary. Molly told her, "Dori, sometimes silence is a no. Sometimes no response from someone is a no. You need to listen to that too. Emily went off to college and she's very busy. She can't talk to you every day like she used to. We'll have to find some other friends for you to talk to." Molly held Dori as she cried.

For young people and adults, friendships and social networks are critical to quality of life and a feeling of connectedness to a community. The social picture of people with ASD and ID in adulthood is rather bleak, with many reporting high levels of loneliness, depression, and dissatisfaction with their social networks (Mazurek, 2014; van Asselt-Goverts et al., 2015).

Research shows that people with ASD and ID also score lower on quality-of-life assessments overall (van Heijst & Geurts, 2015). Some of this is due to limited social and friend networks. People with ID have fewer nondisabled friends than those with physical disabilities, even though people with ID reported participating in more community activities. Most of their social network is made up of caregivers and family members (Lippold & Burns, 2009). One study found that only about half (52%) of older adults with ID had a best friend. A quarter of those with a best friend listed a family member or staff member as their best friend (McCausland et al., 2021).

On a positive note, a literature review found that social skills instruction, informal support, and involvement in support groups increased quality of life for people with ASD (Tobin et al., 2014). People with disabilities deserve well-rounded lives that they feel satisfied with. While social skills are often overlooked as adaptive skills, they have a significant impact on overall quality of life. This book does not address social skills directly, but it would be very difficult to engage in many social activities without the foundational adaptive skills we cover in this book, like listening and responding to verbal interactions, following a routine, and maintaining good hygiene. These are the first place to start building social skills, and many of these are what we call *prerequisite skills,* or skills you need to have first before you can begin to learn a higher-level skill. In practical terms, it can be very hard to make friends if you can't shower, put on deodorant, brush your teeth, and leave the house.

Transition Services

Ben was sure he was ready to work. He had three different internships and four places he regularly volunteered, including his church. He had letters of recommendation, lists of people who would serve as references, a résumé, and a clear idea of what types of jobs he liked: customer service and sales, particularly focused on the outdoors. He had lost count of the number of mock interviews he had completed. What he didn't have was a clear idea of how to make his ideal job, where he wanted to live and how (in an apartment with a roommate), relationships (both friends and romantic), and his finances work out. While most people use the time between high school and adult life to figure these things out, Ben was expected to do this right away once he left high school. He felt very confident about employment, but the rest of the picture was still blank for these other important areas of his life.

Many families do not receive appropriate transition support and planning even though it is required for all students with IEPs. Even students who receive transition services may not leave high school and transition programs with the skills needed to live on their own. Transition supports and services, including vocational rehabilitation, tend to focus primarily on employment outcomes. While future and current employment are important, they are only one piece of the independent living puzzle. Most families are faced with the reality that there are few options for continued services for their child and family, even in the states with the best infrastructure and programming.

The truth is that many students with disabilities graduate or age out of services and their only option is to continue living with their parents for the rest of their lives because they lack the skills to live independently. Many are completely disconnected from services, have no employment or place to go during the day, and very few if any social connections, community involvement, or hobbies. They graduate to their parents' couch. It's one thing if someone chooses to live a life in which they contribute to their family home, take responsibility for household chores, and are active participants in their communities after they graduate or leave school. This may be a wonderful future and exactly what that person and their family wants. The difference in these two situations (staying at home with family because it's what you want versus being forced to stay at home because of lack of options) is *choice*.

Planning for your child's independence now is an excellent first step toward giving them the broadest range of choices in education, employment, living situation, relationships, and anything else you can think of. When we limit a child's independence now by not teaching them the skills they need and fading ourselves (parents and professionals) out of these daily routines, we limit their future choices and options.

Employment

When Esther took her daughter Cam for a job interview at the local gym, she was sure that she and the vocational rehabilitation specialist had planned for everything. Cam was showered and dressed appropriately. She had copies of all her documents, had completed the online application process, and had role-played all the common interview questions. And it went great! Cam got the job!

The initial excitement quickly wore off though, as the real problems didn't start until Cam finished training. She struggled with what to do during "down time" during her shifts, taking directions from bosses she didn't know, and receiving any corrective feedback from her coworkers or boss. One day, she told her regional manager that she wouldn't do one of the main tasks of her job, which was cleaning equipment returned by the gym guests. That was write-up number one. A string of write-ups followed because the more her bosses tried to work with her, the more Cam refused to do the tasks. Esther was beyond exasperated, and then it hit her. This was something Esther couldn't fix. Cam was an adult with a job and the job didn't have to accommodate her. Esther couldn't advocate and help in the ways she used to in high school. There was no IEP team to meet with, no head of special education to petition, and no vocational rehabilitation therapist to intervene. Cam was really on her own to sort this out.

Even when people with disabilities can find employment and maintain a job, there are many barriers to overcome. These include laws and regulations that allow for them to be paid less than minimum wage (yes, that's still legal in many places in the United States; Fair Labor Standards Act, 1938/2008), not to mention unconscious bias or overt discrimination based on their disability (U.S. Equal Employment Opportunity Commission, 2024).

Research has shown that six years after graduation, only between 17 and 39% of adults with ID are employed in competitive integrated settings. Competitive employment means that they competed against typically developing people during the application process and are being paid the standard wage, and integrated means they work alongside typically developing people. Additionally, of those few who are employed, only 59% make more than minimum wage. While there is nothing inherently wrong with a minimum-wage job, minimum wage is not a living wage in most places in the United States. So, what about the rest of the adults with ID? They are either employed in sheltered workshops or in segregated environments away from their typically developing peers, where they make less than minimum wage, or they are completely unemployed (Qian et al., 2018).

People with ASD are even less likely to be employed than those with just ID, with only 25% employed at all and only 6% competitively employed

(Dudley et al., 2015). The good news is that one study found that more independent daily living skills (along with other factors) gave adults with ASD and ID significantly higher likelihood of sustained community employment (Chan et al., 2018).

Independent Living

Kevin, a 28-year-old with autism, was excited to move into his first apartment. He had worked with his family, case manager, state funding programs, and roommate to make this happen, and move-in day was finally here! This was going to put all he had learned about being independent to the test. He'd have to keep his apartment clean, shop for groceries, do his own laundry, and get to work on his own. This means he'd need to use all the strategies for self-management he'd been taught, including breaking big and often overwhelming tasks into bite-sized parts, and then completing them one by one. Both his family and his roommate's family agreed to help them by checking in regularly, especially in the first few weeks as they learned the ropes.

One of Kevin's first obstacles was a common one for someone living with roommates for the first time: dishes left in the sink and taking out the kitchen trash. He'd used his social skills to schedule a time to talk with his roommates, come up with a chore schedule for taking out the trash, and make new rules about the dishes. Crisis averted! Kevin knows there will be other challenges, but he has the support and independent living skills to address them when they come up.

Kevin was very fortunate to have received the training and education he needed to make this big achievement happen. He was also very lucky that his parents encouraged him to do things for himself—he had to admit that while he was learning to do things on his own, he wasn't always so happy about it. In the end, Kevin is glad that his parents insisted that he do things independently. Getting to this place in his life had been so much work, but the excitement he was feeling made it all worth it!

Another area of need for people with ASD and ID is living on their own or with roommates (natural supports). Studies show that by age 23, only between 5 and 19% of young adults with ASD live independently (Forbes et al., 2023; Roux et al., 2015). This is the lowest rate of independent living across disability categories. Conversely, that means between 81 and 95% of this population is living at home with family or in a facility.

One thing that makes living by yourself or with roommates possible is being able to prove financial independence, which is a struggle for people with ASD and ID. They are less likely to have a bank account or credit card, with many remaining under their parents' guardianship, which means they do not have full control of their financial decisions (Human Services Research Institute & National Association of State Directors of Developmental Disabilities Services, 2019; Sanford et al., 2011). The vast majority of those with ASD and ID are also making less than $25,000 a year (Sanford et al., 2011). They may also be limited in how much money they can have in a savings account because it may affect their SSI (supplemental security income) benefits. SSDI (social security disability insurance) also limits how much money a person can gain from work, putting people with disabilities in potentially precarious financial situations.

People with disabilities need as many practice opportunities as possible to learn and maintain skills—so they can earn a living wage, manage their finances, and secure a place to live independently. Starting early and practicing often can help address the deficits in independent living skills that will impact your child's life when they transition into young adulthood, including their ability to hopefully one day live independently.

What's Your Situation?

You've just read snapshots of several families' daily lives. Their stories may be different from or similar to your situation. Some families may be farther down the road than you, but perhaps you can imagine your future self in their shoes, up against the scary statistics of our present moment. The question is, are you willing to work more effectively now to invest in an independent future for your child?

ACTIVITY: Your Efforts

Spend some time pondering the following questions. You may come up with answers as soon as you read them, but spend a day or two thinking about these questions while you are going through daily routines with your child.

Some of your answers may change, or you may see things while engaged in a routine with your child that you didn't think of initially.

- What do your child's morning and bedtime routines look like?
  _____
  _____

- What are the things you have to say and do over and over again to help your child get through the day? _____
  _____

- In what ways do you need to help your child that are above and beyond what you would normally need to do for a neurotypical child? _____
  _____

- How often do you have to be present, just to make sure your child is safe? _____
  _____

ACTIVITY: What If?

Now we'd like you to ponder what would happen (or what likely has already happened) if you were sick in bed. Not sniffles and sneezes, but can't-move-body-ache-fever-misery sick. How would your child fare without you being there in the morning?

	Yes, my child would do this if I did not help them	No, my child would not do this if I did not help them
Would they make it out of bed on time?		
Would they choose school-appropriate clothes to wear?		
Would they choose weather-appropriate clothes to wear to school?		

	Yes, my child would do this if I did not help them	No, my child would not do this if I did not help them
Would they have all the important pieces of clothing on (underwear, shirt, pants/skirt/shorts, socks, and shoes)?		
Would all pieces of clothing be put on correctly (shirt, underwear, and pants/skirt on right-side out and front side forward, and shoes on correct feet)?		
Would they brush their teeth for two minutes using toothpaste?		
Would they wash their face with soap and/or a washcloth?		
Would your child wipe themselves after using the toilet?		
Would they wash their hands thoroughly with soap after using the toilet?		
Would the washing and wiping be done to your standards?		
Would they eat breakfast?		
Would that breakfast be up to your standards for nutrition and meet your child's dietary needs?		

We aren't asking you to contemplate this to upset you, but rather to illustrate the massive degree to which your child relies on you for things as simple as getting dressed and brushing their teeth. Your goal is to teach your child to be more independent. Throughout this book we're going to provide you the knowledge and skills to help support your child as they move toward independence. It will take time, but starting is the first step, and the work gets easier when you stick with it over time. We'll lead you through activities, give you some new vocabulary, and ask you to examine your child's world with a new perspective. Let's get started!

2

"How Am I Supposed to Do This?"
LEVERAGING THE POWER OF TASK ANALYSIS

Jess couldn't believe the statistics she had read in *Spectrum of Independence: How to Teach Your Neurodiverse Child Daily Life Skills*. She knew her son Adam's future would be difficult, but to see the hard numbers on paper just confirmed all her worst fears. She almost tossed the book on the shelf, not wanting to read any more, but then she struck up a conversation with the parent of one of Adam's classmates who happened to also be reading the book. She told Jess that she had continued past that first chapter and was fascinated by the idea of being able to teach her daughter Ava how to complete multistep routines by breaking them down into smaller parts. Although there was a lot of prep work, and the challenge of having to change their deeply ingrained habits was overwhelming at times, she was cautiously optimistic that this could lead to Ava being able to do more things for herself, and smoother mornings and evenings for the entire family. Experiencing newfound hope after her conversation with Ava's mother, Jess was excited to get back to reading the book that night.

The ability to function independently is one of the most important skills a person can have. To live an independent life, a person needs to know how to keep themselves clean, cook, create and follow routines, initiate activities, ask for assistance, self-advocate, and get ready for the day, an event, or bed independently. Your child may be able to learn to perform the tasks needed to get through daily life on their own as an adult. We have seen this happen, and we want nothing more than to show you how to get your child there. Yes, the statistics in Chapter 1 were grim, we admit that. But, as educators, we wouldn't be doing our jobs if we were to leave out what the research shows. The information is meant to shed light on what is likely to happen if proper skills are *not* taught. The good news is that independent-living skills likely *can* be taught to your child! The goal is for your child to live as independently as possible. How? Through the transformational process of task analysis.

Before you begin to learn about task analysis and behavioral interventions, it's important to remember that we will be giving you many new vocabulary words. We will define each of them and we have provided a Glossary in the back of the book for your reference. We use this vocabulary not to confuse you or to sound scientific, but to give you the technical language that your child's IEP team and therapists use. This will allow you to more easily discuss your child's behavior and skills as well as interventions you are using in your home.

What Is Task Analysis?

Task analysis is one of many evidence-based practices that focus on shaping human behavior. For further information about evidence-based practices, take a look at the website of the National Professional Development Center on Autism Spectrum Disorder: *https://autismpdc.fpg.unc.edu*.

The principles of behavioral interventions are based on observing behavior, collecting data to track progress, and developing individualized plans or goals tailored to your child's needs and abilities. When BCBAs say *behavior*, they mean any interaction a person has with their environment that results in a change. Throughout this book we will use the word behavior to refer to both behavior that we want to see (adaptive behavior) or behavior that requires change (challenging or problem behavior). Positive reinforcement like praise or small rewards is used to encourage desired behaviors and to replace challenging ones. Inappropriate behaviors are replaced with more appropriate skills through techniques like modeling and practice. For example, if a child struggles with communication, using these principles can help teach them to express their needs using words or gestures.

In addition to positive reinforcement, other key tools include prompting, chaining, and systematically fading prompts. Prompts provide helpful cues to guide your child through a step of a process or skill. You will learn all about using prompts to teach in Chapter 6. Chaining involves linking together individual steps that were learned separately, which you'll learn about in Chapter 7. Fading prompts entails gradually decreasing the number and intensity of prompts, which we'll cover in Chapter 8.

Task analysis is the main teaching method we'll be covering in this book. A task analysis involves methodically breaking down a routine into manageable parts so that you can pinpoint which part of the sequence is causing a problem. A *routine* is a multistep activity that achieves a final outcome. You likely engage in numerous routines a day, from getting ready in the morning and showering to mealtimes. A routine can be simple or quite complicated. For example, you might consider washing dishes to be a single activity, but for children with disabilities, it's a routine with many small steps, such as putting soap on the sponge, turning the faucet on, wetting the sponge, and more. You will begin to see how seemingly simple tasks like putting on a jacket are really multistep routines.

The task analysis process allows skills to be taught incrementally and systematically, starting with the simplest of actions. The skills are built over time, usually getting easier and going more quickly, until full mastery of the larger routine is achieved. We will share examples of this process later in this chapter. Data are recorded throughout this process to track progress and give you the information you need to make adjustments when warranted.

Numerous research studies spanning decades have proven the effectiveness of evidence-based practices in developing communication and social skills, improving academic ability, teaching vocational skills, and of course increasing daily living abilities (adaptive skills) in children with autism and other developmental disorders (Wong et al., 2015). Skills learned through the use of evidence-based practices lead to greater independence and improved quality of life.

You might be thinking that this sounds like a really promising way to help your child increase their independence. We agree—with one caveat: It takes work! Just like with any new skill, it takes time before the new skill becomes a habit for your child. And consistency on your part is key. But if you are willing to apply these principles systematically and consistently, as we will teach you how to do step by step, you can help your child replace prompt-dependent skills with independent skills.

What Tasks Should Be Broken Down?

Any routine that is needed to get through the day—that is, any routine necessary for independent living—is a good candidate for task analysis. A more comprehensive list is included in Chapter 7, but here is a snapshot of a just a few everyday routines that you might consider:

- Washing hands
- Brushing teeth
- Undressing
- Getting dressed
- Showering
- Preparing a simple meal
- Cleaning a bedroom
- Doing laundry

As your child masters these skills, task analysis can be applied to more advanced routines, such as choosing something healthy to eat, prioritizing necessary activities over preferred activities, initiating an activity with another person, or creating a schedule. Evidence-based practices like prompting and task analyses are versatile, and can be applied to just about any routine.

How Are Routines Broken Down?

You'll learn how to analyze the routine and break it down into microsteps in Chapter 7. Here's a sneak peek of what a task analysis for taking off shoes looks like.

- Sit down on the floor
- Untie shoelaces on left foot
- Put right hand on left heel
- Push shoe off
- Place shoe on floor
- Untie shoelaces on right shoe
- Put left hand on right heel
- Push shoe off

- Place shoe on floor
- Stand up
- Pick up shoes
- Put shoes away

Bet you never considered how complex this routine is, huh? To you, this is just one quick, simple action that you may be able to do without consciously thinking about it. To your child, it is a complicated, multistep process. If your child struggles with one of the microsteps, the remaining steps can't be accomplished, and the task doesn't get completed. Your job in this book will be to determine where in the process your child needs help, and then you'll learn how to teach that skill or modify the activity so that they can complete the activity as independently as possible.

What Is Expected of Me?

When we work with families, we see how much they are up against. You're likely in the same boat and eager for solutions. We're eager to give them to you. But know that our solutions aren't a quick fix—they will take time and effort, and a willingness to work with your child in a different way. What you have been doing isn't working, or hasn't been as effective as you'd like, which is why you've picked up this book. We know you've been doing your best. Possibly you have been parenting your child the same way you parent your typically developing children, but without the same results. We'll show you a different way of supporting your child with an intellectual or developmental disability—and how to teach them new skills that will last a lifetime.

So, what does all of this work entail? Here's a general overview of what you'll be expected to do:

- Honestly assess your child's readiness to learn independent living skills (Chapter 3)
- Honestly assess your own readiness to teach independent living skills using task analysis (Chapter 4)
- Be consistent (every chapter!)
- Identify an initial routine you want to target (Chapter 7)
- Record data (this chapter)

- Use prompts skillfully (Chapter 6)
- Create a task analysis (Chapter 7)
- Fade (or remove) prompts wisely (Chapter 8)
- Differentiate between modifications and accommodations (Chapter 9)

We know this sounds like a lot. But your follow-through is absolutely crucial to your child's success now and in the future. It can help to keep in mind that learning how to do all these things is an investment in both your child's future, as well as yours.

Tracking Data

As a parent of a child with disabilities, you've probably had it up to here with being asked about or talked to about data. We get it. Parenting is an extreme sport, and you're busy. There are exceptional emotional highs and devastating lows, and sometimes those two things happen within minutes of each other. That is part of parenting. However, these highs and lows can have a significant impact on how you feel about your child's abilities and performance and your hopes and thoughts about their future.

Data, on the other hand, are impartial. Luckily for us, the data don't care what type of day you're having. Data don't know if you're annoyed, tired, or on top of the world. Data are data. The data you collect will allow you to see the objective truth about your child's abilities and performance unattached from your current mood or situation.

This level of objectivity can be a saving grace. On a good day, you can look at the data and feel proud that you've made progress fading your assistance, and that your child is getting closer to his goal. On a hard day, you can look at those very same data and see objectively that your child has, in fact, made progress in spite of what the fatalistic voice in your head might be telling you. Hard days will happen, and having robust data can help you stave off feelings of overwhelm ("I can't keep doing this"), catastrophizing ("He won't ever learn!"), or overgeneralizing ("Nothing works!"). These thoughts can get the best of anyone, and it's good to have data as a safeguard against your own potential anxiety and doubts.

As an additional bonus, behavior data can be used for other purposes. The data can be presented during IEP meetings in school to show your child's progress. They can confirm or refute assertions that your child has not made progress. Data can also be given to behavior specialists or other professionals who may come to work with your child at home or at school, to show the effectiveness of the interventions you are already using. Data can also help you decide when a goal is mastered or needs to be taught differently due to lack of progress. The data may also be helpful to professionals like occupational and physical therapists who want to see how your child uses their skills in the natural environment, and what skills may need to be targeted to increase their independence during daily living activities. For example, if your occupational therapist can see that your child is having trouble with the specific step of grasping their toothbrush, or the physical therapist can see that your child is struggling with balance when putting on pants while standing up, coordination when lining up the zipper on their jacket, or strength to lift the jug of orange juice to pour, they can create plans and suggest exercises to address these needs. By pinpointing exactly where in the routine your child is experiencing problems, other specialists can be called in to support as needed.

So how much data are we asking you to track? We're keeping it simple. All you'll need to track are the type and frequency of the prompts you're giving to your child. That's it. Blank data sheets will be provided later in the book, so all you'll need to do is note which type of support you provide your child and make tally marks for the number of prompts you give. You can see examples of filled-out and blank data sheets at *www.guilford.com/lombardi-forms*.

Now, taking data can be difficult if you're trying to avoid getting soap everywhere while your child washes their hands, or keeping the peanut butter mostly in the jar while they make themselves toast. This is why we're not asking you to make check marks while wrangling your whole crew in the morning.

Instead, we strongly suggest taking your data *after* the routine is done. Now, you won't be able to do this from memory, so you'll want to record the routine on your phone or another smart device. You'll play back these videos and use the data sheets to document what kind of help you're providing to your child, any prompts you may be giving to your child, and what parts of the routine your child is doing by themselves. These snippets of your child's day will help you examine the routines you choose to target down to minute details.

A couple tips, first, you may need to play around with the angles and where you place your camera; an inexpensive tripod can be a good investment. Second, if your child is distracted by the camera, tell them they can watch it later; some kids really like watching themselves on the phone screen. You can even point out to them what parts of the routine they're doing by themselves with some fanfare!

How often will you need to record data? Since we're focused on independent living routines that take place anywhere from five times a week (getting home from school) to 21 times a week (mealtimes), and you are choosing one routine at a time, we're very hopeful that you can take data on that routine between two and five times a week. If taking data between two and five times a week does not seem feasible, we'll give you some ideas for ways to get time back in Chapter 4. Taking data is an important part of this process. Being able to review your child's progress can be very rewarding.

Giving Directions Rather Than Suggestions

Parents will often say to their child, "Why don't we go upstairs and take a bath?" or "What about wearing the clean shirt instead?" when they really mean, "Walk upstairs and get ready for your bath" and "Put on the clean shirt." Does this sound familiar? No one wants to be seen as a dictator, so we learn to request things politely. We position directives as suggestions so the other person feels as if they have a choice. Adults understand this nuance. Children don't. All they hear is a question—a question that leaves the choice up to them.

But some things simply aren't up for discussion. Activities of daily living are nonnegotiable. Teeth simply have to be brushed, meals must be eaten, and shoes are required to go most places in public. These things aren't optional no matter how much your child (and maybe you also) might wish they were. So, you'll need to be fully on board with giving directives rather than suggestions going forward until your child can self-start these routines.

Realize that telling your child exactly what to do (and not do) provides structure. When we say structure, we don't mean it has to be rigid, only that you are providing your child a framework for how the world works. Certain things must be done in life, end of story. If that framework is up for debate or missing altogether, your child will have a harder time distinguishing must-dos from maybes, and that can impact their ability to live independently. If you can do this, you're much more likely to be successful with this program.

Motivating with Reinforcement

Motivation to complete a task is often related to how much or what kind of *reinforcement* is available. Reinforcement is receiving something that you prefer (or the removal of something you dislike) that is presented (or removed) after a behavior. Think of it like this, most of us go to work at least partially for the paycheck, which makes it worth our while to be there. Our job doesn't give us the paycheck before we go to work and get our job duties done. For all of us, using reinforcement can help with motivation. This is not the same as a bribe. Bribes get paid before the behavior we want to see (as in, "If I give you this sticker, will you sit nicely for the doctor?"). Reinforcement happens after (as in, "You did a great job in the doctor's appointment! Go pick a sticker from the treasure box!"). It's well-documented in research that providing *positive reinforcement* after your child performs a specific task or set of tasks increases the likelihood that your child will do those tasks again in the future.

Reinforcement is a powerful tool for changing and shaping behaviors. Put simply, reinforcement is something that happens after a behavior that increases the likelihood of that behavior happening again. Reinforcement can help your child take a more active interest in their independent living routines. For some routines, the reinforcement is built in. When you make an after-school snack, the reinforcement is clear. You make the snack; you get to eat the snack. Getting to eat the snack makes you more likely to do the behavior of making the snack in the future, or said another way, being allowed to eat the snack *reinforces* the behavior of making the snack.

Reinforcement could also take the form of verbal praise ("Great job finishing your homework!") or access to a preferred activity or item (time to play, watching a favorite show) in the hope that they'll do it again. In order to be successful in this program, you will need to accept the responsibility of using positive reinforcement with your child—and being consistent! There are many types of reinforcement that are discussed in more detail in Chapter 5. For now, it is only important that you be on board with using reinforcement as generously as is needed in the initial stages of learning to get your child to a level where they do not need continuous reinforcement to stay on task.

Excited yet? We hope you are! Our goal in presenting the research in

Chapter 1 was to give you the answer to "Why" you should increase your child's independence. The goal of Chapter 2 was to give you insight into "How" you can increase independence. Answering the first question will give you the motivation you need to help your child become more independent, and answering the second question will give you the tools that you will use to do it. Having that clear in your head, let's move on to Part II of the book—assessment.

Part II

Assessment

3

"Is My Child Ready for This?"
EVALUATING YOUR CHILD'S READINESS

Lisa walked down the driveway and waited for the school bus to drop off her three children from school, wondering how the afternoon routine always felt so out of hand. Once 10-year-old Chris, 7-year-old Jack, and 5-year-old Laura got off the school bus, they all walked back up the driveway. All three children were diagnosed with autism; however, they were three entirely different kids. Chris was in a fifth-grade inclusion class, fully verbal, and capable of completing some tasks independently—although he frequently looked for assistance as a way to get attention or just flat-out didn't seem interested in doing a task. Jack, on the other hand, was in a self-contained class, had limited language, and required a lot more supervision than the other two. Laura was in a self-contained kindergarten class. Although her language was delayed, she was able to communicate and generally followed directions in familiar routines.

It was a beautiful day outside. As they walked into the house, Lisa told the kids they could play in the backyard after Chris finished his homework and she finished a few things for work. This part of the afternoon was very stressful, and Lisa constantly felt like she needed four of her to get through the afternoon—one for each child and one to finish her work. Chris walked into the mudroom, promptly took off his jacket and shoes, and dropped them on the floor on top of his backpack before running into the kitchen. Lisa first helped Jack hang up his backpack and watched him take off his shoes and put them in the closet, while Laura stood there and waited for Lisa to help her. Next, she helped Lisa take her shoes off, hang up her jacket, and put her backpack on the high hook she couldn't reach. Then she called Chris back to the mudroom to hang up his jacket, put his shoes away, and bring his backpack into the kitchen so she could empty it and see what he had for homework. Instead of coming back to the mudroom, he started whining that he needed help. In the interest of time and so she could get back to her work, Lisa ended up hanging up his jacket for him and carrying his backpack into the kitchen. He then had another thing to whine about because Lisa told him that he couldn't have cookies for a snack. After the kids finished eating, they went into the den to watch a show and play with their toys. Lisa headed into the adjoining room to finish up a few things in her home office. She knew getting Chris away from the television to do his homework was going to be a fight, especially because Jack and Laura were allowed to stay and watch television as they did not get any homework.

When Lisa stepped out of her office five minutes later, Jack was not in the den anymore. She asked Chris where he was, but engrossed in the television, Chris just ignored her. Laura played with her favorite toy and sang a song quietly to herself. Lisa didn't panic, but she was immediately worried. Jack had a history of eloping (leaving safe areas and people), and she knew she needed to act fast. She saw him running around in the front of the house, which she had told him over and over wasn't safe. She called him from the front door, hoping he would run back inside. When he did not come to the door, Lisa headed out to get him. As she approached him, she started to scold him for running out of the house alone and without his shoes. She quickly realized he also had something in his mouth. She put her hand out and he promptly spit out a chewed-up piece of cardboard that he must have ripped off a game box in the den closet. Although Lisa longed for the day when Jack did not require constant supervision, she had to remind herself that today was not that day.

Now that you have a general idea of what's involved in this program, the first step is to assess whether your child is ready for it. While this book is intended to work for most families with a neurodiverse child, not every child with a developmental or intellectual disability will find success with this program. Some children, especially those with physical limitations or a history of engaging in unsafe behaviors, may need the support of other professionals like behavior analysts, occupational therapists, and physical therapists. Other children may simply not be ready, and first need to focus on learning foundational skills. This chapter will help you determine if your child is prepared to safely and productively participate in this program. It is divided into two sections:

- **Unsafe behaviors** (behavior we do *not* want your child to be engaging in): These are behaviors that would greatly increase the risk of injury to your child or others, such as hitting or leaving safe areas and adults.
- **Foundational skills** (behaviors we *do* want your child to be engaging in): These are prerequisite skills that your child should be able to complete independently, such as the ability to follow directions.

The material presented in this chapter will either give you the go-ahead to move forward with the activities in the book, or direct you to resources to address any unsafe behaviors or missing skills in your child's repertoire.

Is There a Medical Reason for Your Child's Behavior?

The very first thing a behavior specialist or any professional should have you assess for is a medical reason for your child's behavior. For example, a child with recurrent ear infections may not be ignoring you but rather experiencing temporary hearing loss. A child who is crying and rubbing their eyes and nose suddenly may have an illness or allergy. A child who has frequent tantrums may be in pain. Medical reasons for behavior should be addressed by the appropriate medical professional before behavioral intervention planning takes place. Please be sure to rule out medical reasons for problem behavior first!

Unsafe Behaviors

Sometimes children and adolescents with developmental delays engage in dangerous behaviors. This may be due to having a limited ability to communicate, low impulse control, low frustration tolerance, or a lack of understanding of the natural consequences of engaging in a certain behavior. For example, if I run away from my family, I may get lost. They may also engage in dangerous sensory-seeking behaviors such as head banging or pulling out their hair.

Sometimes, even with the best of intentions, families give in, or reward their child's unsafe or escalating behavior. This leads to the child learning that sometimes, if not all the time, certain behaviors get them what they want (if I hit my brother, he will drop the toy and I can play with it; if I bang my head on the floor, my mom will leave me alone and not make me brush my teeth). Of course, it may be necessary at times to appease your child in the short term, for the sake of everyone's safety; however, long term, you want your child to learn appropriate replacement behaviors so they don't need to engage in problem behavior to get what they want.

The list of behaviors that follows is particularly dangerous within the context of this program, because the goal of this program is to eventually remove yourself from your child's presence during these routines. If your child cannot be safe on their own to complete these tasks, then you must remain with them to keep them safe.

Let's look at how safety factors into a common scenario. Imagine it's a weekday, and your child decides midway through getting dressed for school that he wants to watch a show in his underwear. You need to know that if something like that were to happen, you could redirect him back to his room to finish getting dressed *without fear of him engaging in a behavior that could lead to a tantrum or injuries.* In addition, you need to be confident that once you reach the part of the program where you increase your distance, your child *will not engage in a dangerous behavior when they are left alone to complete the routine.* Using the example above, you would need to be confident that if you left your child in his room to get dressed while you went to your room to get dressed, you would not look through your bedroom window and see him running down the driveway headed for the busy street.

Being Safe versus Behaving Safely

If you are thinking, "Phew! My child would never run into traffic! And she doesn't engage in any of the unsafe behaviors discussed so far in this chapter," then she may be ready to begin this program. However—and this is important—if you walk on eggshells around your child, making sure that everything is exactly as they want it so that they don't have a "need" to engage in unsafe behaviors, how certain can you be that they have good safety skills? This is the difference between attempting to create a safe environment for your child so that they can *be safe* versus knowing that your child will *behave safely* in the natural environment. You want to know without a doubt that when your child is asked to do nonpreferred activities, has to wait for a preferred activity, is redirected back to a task, or is given limited supervision, they will not engage in unsafe behaviors.

For example, if you are in the habit of never leaving small items lying around the house because your child is likely to ingest them, you have attempted to create a safe environment. This is in comparison to a situation with a child who could come across a small item and not have any interest in ingesting the item. If you have doubts, refer to the Help! section of any behaviors that are of concern, and follow the guidance there before beginning this program.

Self-Injurious Behavior

DESCRIPTION: Any occurrence where the child attempts to harm or succeeds in harming themselves is self-injurious behavior. These actions are typically categorized as either *socially mediated behavior* or *sensory mediated behavior*. With socially mediated behavior, your child is looking for a reaction from you or others to gain something or to avoid something. With sensory mediated behavior, your child is meeting an internal sensory need, and the presence of others has no bearing on whether he engages in the behavior (that is, he would do the same behavior alone in his room as he would in front of you). The important thing to keep in mind is that it does not matter if your child is engaging in these behaviors to communicate frustration or for sensory reasons—both are considered unsafe.

EXAMPLES: Head banging; biting themselves; hitting themselves (anywhere on their body); punching themselves; picking skin or sores; excessive rubbing or scratching of any body parts/skin; poking/gouging themselves, especially in the eyes, ears, or other soft-tissue areas; sticking fingers or objects down their throats to induce vomiting.

SCENARIOS:

1. Your child is playing video games instead of finishing their homework. When told that they need to finish their homework, they begin biting their arm and looking at you for a reaction. This is an example of an unsafe socially mediated behavior.
2. Your child is alone in the living room, happily watching their favorite movie. They are also biting their arm. This is an example of an unsafe sensory mediated behavior.

WHY IT'S DANGEROUS: Engagement in these behaviors is dangerous for obvious reasons—you don't want your child to hurt themselves. In connection to this program, as mentioned, you need to be able to safely and confidently redirect your child during a task sequence or routine, without worrying that they will engage in self-injurious behavior. Then later, when you fade yourself out of the routines, you need to be confident that your child won't self-harm or put themselves in a dangerous situation when you are not present.

QUESTIONS TO ASK YOURSELF:

- Does my child engage in any of the self-injurious behaviors listed?
- Does my child hurt or attempt to hurt themselves when there is a known reason including being told to do something difficult, a change in routine, or denial or delay to access activity/item?
- Does my child hurt or attempt to hurt themselves if there is no known reason (sensory, internal, or when they are alone)?
- Does my child engage in a behavior that could cause them harm even if it has not yet (the child hits themselves in the head but does not create bruises or red marks)?

HELP! MY CHILD ENGAGES IN SELF-INJURIOUS BEHAVIOR: Self-injurious behaviors can be difficult to stop. Your safest option is to hire a behavior analyst to help you or to advocate for your school-based team to provide you with behaviorally based family training at home. A professional can help you to understand why your child is engaging in these behaviors (or confirm that your theories are correct) through assessments and observations, and help you put a function-based plan in place to safely address these behaviors. If no one is available to come to you in person (often true for folks who live in rural areas or certain states), seek out a behavior analyst who can help you virtually by using telehealth or online supports.

Now, some parents feel that seeking professional help will undermine their ability to intuitively parent their child. If this is your concern, please know that we are big believers in a parent's expertise in their own child—a parent knows their child best, is their child's biggest advocate, and is their only lifelong teacher. However, we are also equally big believers in reducing parents' daily struggles in raising a child with a developmental or intellectual disability—it is not always easy, and sometimes the solutions aren't as commonsense as we'd hope.

If the professional is well trained, they may be able to offer insights and ideas you have not considered. Sometimes, just having an objective perspective can be helpful. For example, a parent makes a general comment to her three children who are watching TV to clean up their toys. The neurotypical children start to clean up, but the child with autism continues to play. The parent thinks the child is being defiant. A behavior analyst may point out that their child likely did not process the direction because they were too engaged in the television show; the parent realizes that next time she should try turning off the television to see if that helps get her child's attention before asking the child to clean the room. A fresh perspective can lead to a greater understanding of the situation and to a more effective solution—without the stress.

Aggressive Behaviors

DESCRIPTION: Aggressive behavior is any behavior that is directed at other people that has the potential to cause physical harm.

EXAMPLES: Biting, hitting, slapping, scratching, kicking, spitting, head butting, pinching, hair pulling, throwing objects at someone.

SCENARIOS:

1. You ask your child to come inside and he verbally protests. When you repeat yourself, he starts to hit and kick you.
2. You tell your child she cannot have cookies before dinner, and she starts to scratch you.

WHY IT'S DANGEROUS: Any time a child attempts to harm another person, you run the risk of someone getting hurt—whether it is the person being physically hurt, or the child who is now in a position of being blocked, restrained, or otherwise contained. Also, as a child gets older, they get bigger . . . and stronger. This can lead to more dangerous outcomes when they become aggressive, including run-ins with law enforcement. The earlier you can address this type of behavior, the better.

QUESTIONS TO ASK YOURSELF:

- Does my child attempt to or succeed in physically harming me or others in the vicinity if he is mad or upset?
- Will my child resort to aggression if other behaviors do not get him what he wants?

HELP! MY CHILD ENGAGES IN AGGRESSIVE BEHAVIOR: Similar to self-injurious behaviors, aggressive behaviors can be dangerous and difficult to stop. They also require a multifaceted approach that involves a combination of removing reinforcement for the aggressive behavior and steps to teach replacement behaviors. See the Help! section for self-injurious behaviors for more information about the benefits of hiring a professional for additional guidance.

Elopement (Leaving Safe Areas or Safe People)

DESCRIPTION: Any time a child runs away from an adult or moves out of an assigned area, it is considered elopement.

EXAMPLES: Children could be looking for the thrill of the chase, just taking off to explore, or trying to get away from demands or unpleasant sensory input. No matter the why, it is all considered eloping.

SCENARIOS:

1. A child takes off running, and then checks back over their shoulder to see if anyone is chasing them. They might be laughing and having a good time while doing this. This might be socially mediated elopement.
2. You are at an amusement park and your child keeps running up ahead

of the group without realizing that they are not with the group. They are not running for the thrill of the chase, they are just taking off to explore. When you catch up to them, they are unaware that they were ever in danger of losing the group. This is automatically mediated elopement.
3. A child who does not like showering runs out of the bathroom when their parent turns on the water. This is another example of socially mediated elopement.

WHY IT'S DANGEROUS: The more space you give them, the farther they could run off before you have realized. During the routines we cover in this book, your child will need to eventually complete them on their own. Elopement can be a huge safety risk, so your child cannot be left alone to complete these routines. You want your child to be aware of their surroundings and have the impulse control to stay in a designated area of their own accord (not because they are gated or blocked in).

QUESTIONS TO ASK YOURSELF:
- Does my child take off running and want to be chased?
- If I am engaged with my child with an activity, do we need to be in a contained area for my child to stay with me?
- If my child is engaged in a nonpreferred activity at home, do they require redirection to remain in the area until the activity is complete (eating dinner at the table)?

HELP! MY CHILD ELOPES: To do this program, you must feel secure that your child will stay engaged in a preferred activity (watching a movie), and ideally a nonpreferred activity (brushing teeth) too, without running off. If you answered "yes" to the above questions, your homework is to teach your child to independently stay in a designated area. A great parent-friendly resource on this topic is Mark Durand's *Optimistic Parenting*. If your child has ever left your home or gone into an unsafe area in your home (a woodshop, attic, or unfinished basement), you may need the support of a professional like a behavior analyst to assess the function of the behavior, design an intervention, and support you in implementing the intervention to keep your child safe.

Pica (Eating Nonfood Items)

DESCRIPTION: *Pica* is a disorder where a person compulsively eats items that are not food and that do not have any nutritional value.

EXAMPLES: People with pica will ingest things such as dirt, shampoo, small toys, paper, and cardboard. Any item that is not food is a possibility, but some people with pica have preferences for the types of materials they will eat (they could eat string or cloth, but not metal objects).

SCENARIOS:

1. While outside playing, your daughter picks up a rock and puts it in her mouth.
2. While in the bathroom, your son tries to drink the shampoo.

WHY IT'S DANGEROUS: Ingesting nonedible items can cause major medical issues such as toxic poisoning, stomach or intestinal ruptures, stomach or intestinal blockages, or incessant vomiting.

QUESTIONS TO ASK YOURSELF:

- Do I need to keep a close eye on my child to make sure they do not ingest any nonfood items?
- Do I worry that my child may try to eat nonfood items if left unsupervised, in a nonsecure room?
- Have I found my child with nonedible things in his mouth?

HELP! MY CHILD ENGAGES IN PICA: Sometimes children engage in pica because they are lacking needed minerals. Speak to your child's pediatrician to determine whether your child may be deficient in any minerals. Once that is ruled out, we recommend working with a professional like a behavior analyst with experience specifically in treating pica. There is research on effective interventions, but these interventions require parents to be trained by a professional.

Property Destruction

DESCRIPTION: *Property destruction* is defined as damaging personal or public property.

EXAMPLES: Throwing or kicking items, ripping or breaking items, swiping items off a table, dumping bins, ripping items off walls.

SCENARIOS:

1. You ask your child to do their homework and they throw a container of pencils across the room.
2. You ask your child to share their toys with their cousin and they break one of the toys.

WHY IT'S DANGEROUS: Punching a wall, kicking furniture, breaking glass, or any other form of property destruction can lead to injuries to both the child and the parent attempting to block or redirect.

QUESTIONS TO ASK YOURSELF:

- Does my child destroy things when they do not get their way?
- Do I worry that my child will throw an item if they get upset?
- Do I keep things put away, off the tables, and so on out of fear that my child will have more items to throw, rip, swipe, or break if they get upset?

HELP! MY CHILD ENGAGES IN PROPERTY DESTRUCTION: This behavior needs an approach with a combination of removing reinforcement for the dangerous behavior, while simultaneously teaching replacement behaviors. For example, you want your child to know that any mess they make will result in them needing to clean it up and that they will still have to do the task they were avoiding. You may need to ensure a loss of access to certain toys or items until your child has demonstrated that they can be safe with those items. Additionally, teach your child how to request a break, communicate their feelings with words, and do deep breathing or other calming strategies proactively, with the goal of replacing the destructive behavior with more appropriate behavior.

Inability to Self-Regulate
(Inability for the Child to Calm Down Once Upset)

DESCRIPTION: The ability to *self-regulate* means that once upset, a child can calm themselves down (or calm down with minimal support from another person), within a reasonable amount of time.

EXAMPLES: Lacking this skill shows up as a child's inability to self-soothe, leading to a prolonged state of dysregulation, escalation to a state of extreme distress, or engagement in dangerous behaviors (as in self-injury, aggression, or property destruction).

SCENARIOS:

1. Your child is denied iPad time before bed and begins to whine and cry. Any attempts by you to either talk to them, redirect them, or ignore them results in an increase in the intensity of the behaviors, usually to the point of a full-out tantrum that continues for more than five minutes. It may escalate to the point of self-injurious or aggressive behavior.
2. Your child's toy just broke. He gets mildly upset but brings the toy to you and asks you to fix it. When you can't fix it, he spirals into a full-blown tantrum that lasts several minutes.

WHY IT'S DANGEROUS: When a child can't self-regulate, others run the risk of triggering behaviors that could escalate into dangerous behaviors and carry on for an excessive amount of time. You may also feel the need to walk on eggshells out of fear of setting off a behavior, which is a stressful way to parent. Another risk is that, in an attempt to calm your child, you may give them what they initially asked for like the iPad or something similarly off-limits like your phone. This only teaches the child that tantrums get you to meet their demands. It doesn't teach them to calm down on their own, find other activities to do, or how to self-soothe during an upsetting situation.

QUESTIONS TO ASK YOURSELF:

- When my child gets upset, does it take more than five minutes for him to calm down?
- When upset, does my child's behavior escalate, sometimes to the point of self-injurious or aggressive behavior?
- Does my child's behavior escalate if I speak to or redirect him when upset?
- Does my child resist redirection to another item or activity if he is upset?
- Do I need to give in to the initial demand for him to calm down?

HELP! MY CHILD CANNOT REGULATE THEIR EMOTIONS: If you answered "yes" to any of these questions, your child is not able to self-regulate. This is a common issue for children with developmental delays. You may find that it is helpful to consult a behavior analyst or other professional to create a plan and support you as you navigate this behavior.

ACTIVITY: Child Behavior Safety Assessment

Now let's determine where your child might be on the safety spectrum by completing the following assessment. Please read through the list of behaviors in the table below and check "yes" or "no" based on whether your child exhibits these behaviors *within your home*. Please complete this assessment based on situations where your child is being asked to do nonpreferred tasks, has the freedom to leave the designated area, and is not being bribed, coaxed, or promised something they love for completing the activity. Given the severity of the consequences of the behaviors listed, it is particularly important that you adopt an objective and honest perspective on your child's current safety skills.

Behavior	YES, my child does engage in this behavior	NO, my child does not engage in this behavior
Self-injurious behavior		
Physical aggression toward others		
Elopement		
Pica		
Property destruction		

Behavior	NO, my child cannot do this	YES, my child can do this
Self-regulation		

That being said, if your child only engages in a behavior in very specific, controllable situations, you can score that as a "no." For example, if the only nonedible thing your child eats is Play-Doh, and your child does not have access to Play-Doh in your house, then you can check "no" for "pica." If your child has a history of ingesting nonedible items that you cannot clear from your home, then you would check "yes" for "pica." Engagement in these behaviors outside of the home only does not constitute a "yes." We are concerned specifically with behaviors that your child engages in inside your home.

SCORING

If you checked the column on the right for all behaviors, you have cleared this hurdle! However, if you marked any behaviors in the left column, then you will need to address those behaviors before beginning this program, or consider that this program may not be a good fit for your child. You may be able to address any behavioral issues with guidance from self-help books or online resources, or you may find that you need to consult with a professional.

Foundational Skills

Once you have ascertained that your child does not have any behaviors that could be safety concerns, the next step is to determine if they have certain foundational learning skills or *prerequisite skills.* Learning skills encompass a variety of areas, all of which contribute to a child being teachable. These skills include things such as the ability to independently sit or stand at a table or some other assigned area, the ability to pay attention to a parent or therapist, willingness to engage in presented tasks, willingness to participate in adult-directed activities, and the ability to accept redirection and prompts when they are unable to complete a task independently.

The presence of these skills leads to more productive teaching and a greater likelihood of success with this program. If these skills are not present, they can be taught; however, they are generally best taught in controlled situations, usually at a table and using a method like discrete trial teaching. Discrete trial teaching is outside the scope of this book, but it is an evidence-based practice that many behavior therapists and some special education teachers use in their practice. Once the skills are mastered in a controlled environment with direct teaching, they can be generalized out into the natural environment and eventually into a multistep daily living routine.

There are several reasons for introducing these skills in a controlled environment. For one, there are fewer distractions in a controlled environment; when in the natural environment, bath toys in the tub may be a distraction during handwashing, or snack foods in the kitchen may grab a child's attention while emptying their backpack. Another reason is that although the completion of a routine may be rewarding, the routines in and of themselves are not generally enjoyable; as the routines are composed of multiple parts, reinforcement is generally delayed until the completion of the routine. For instance, you don't get to drink the smoothie until you're done making it. Finally, the completion of the morning or nighttime routine is usually time-sensitive, only adding to the stress; the time-sensitive nature of the morning and nighttime routines limits your ability as a parent to see your child through to the end of the task if they engage in any off-task behaviors during the process. All of these issues can be eliminated when teaching skills in a controlled environment.

The Importance of Learning to Follow Directions

Remember: If your goal is to prepare your child for an inclusive higher education program, competitive and integrated employment, or independent living, their ability to take direction and handle tasks they don't want to do will be important. This is just as important for neurotypical folks too! Put simply, your child will be directed by people (both adults and peers) their entire life, so it's important to have a foundation of those interactions. As authors, we were directed by our editors to make multiple rounds of edits for our book. No, the edits weren't fun, but they were still important.

Let's briefly look at adult-directed tasks in the life of a neurodiverse child. When a child starts school—whether it is special education or general education—the teacher directs the class. This starts as early as nursery school. The nursery school teacher is not asking little three-year-old Johnny what he would like to do all day. The teacher announces to the class that it is circle time and Johnny is expected to sit on the carpet, with everyone else, and attend to the lesson—whether he wants to or not. This setup, with a few modifications, continues through high school.

Let's jump forward to college. Some students are fortunate enough to get accepted into an inclusive higher education program. Inclusive higher education programs provide access to the college experience for students with intellectual disability. Although students who enter these programs participate in creating their schedule and choosing some of their classes, they also have required classes and activities. If Johnny does not want to take a required course, he won't complete the program.

Now let's assume that Johnny has finished college and has a job. At work, he is expected to perform all the duties associated with that position. He is being paid, and he does not have an aide or job coach with him at work. Johnny won't get to decide what he wants to do all day when he is at work. This is a real job, in the real world, with real expectations.

Johnny finishes up his workday and heads home. He has his own apartment and lives with a roommate. At this point his activities become self-directed, as there's no authority figure or aide reminding him what needs to get done. This is where the core foundational life skills that he learned in childhood come into play. As a boy, Johnny was taught by adults to complete nonpreferred activities before engaging in preferred activities. By the time he became a young adult, he had developed the self-direction and self-restraint to engage in nonpreferred activities like food shopping, cooking, and cleaning his home *before* engaging in preferred activities like hanging out with his friends or watching television.

None of us live in a world where we get to do whatever we want all day. We all have responsibilities that can be viewed as nonpreferred tasks. We all have rules and directives that we need to follow. Have you renewed your driver's license lately? Or filed your taxes? Most people find those tasks to be pretty nonpreferred. We all have times when we would prefer not to complete a task in that moment, but we would experience pretty big consequences if we did not. We need to get dressed in the morning and go to work, even if we would prefer to stay home in our sweatpants and scroll on our phone; otherwise, we risk losing our job. We all have to follow the speed limit laws when we drive or risk getting a ticket.

Given this perspective, please keep in mind that although many of the foundational skills involve the completion of nonpreferred tasks, that does not make them any less important. In fact, in many cases, these skills are some of the most important things you can teach your child for them to be successful later in life.

Engagement in Preferred Activities

DESCRIPTION: The ability to stay on task and complete an enjoyable activity without needing support from others. Such activities are categorized as being either *open-ended*, meaning they do not have a definitive end, or *closed-ended*, meaning they have a definitive end point. It doesn't matter if the activities are open-ended or closed-ended, only that they are preferred.

SCENARIOS:

1. Your child loves to play with their action figurines, and if left in the living room with their toys, they would stay in the area and play with their toys appropriately for at least five minutes. This is an example of staying on task during an open-ended activity.
2. Your child loves puzzles, and if left alone at the kitchen table with a puzzle, they would stay in the area until the puzzle was completed. This is an example of staying on task during a closed-ended activity.

WHY IT'S IMPORTANT: The ability to stay on task during a preferred activity requires a certain level of self-control and ability to sustain attention, albeit at a lower level than would be required to stay on task during a nonpreferred activity. Therefore, staying on task during a preferred activity is usually a prerequisite for staying on task during a nonpreferred activity.

QUESTIONS TO ASK YOURSELF:

- Does my child have activities that they enjoy?
- Is my child able to play with toys appropriately?

- If my child engages in *stereotypic behavior* (a repetitive behavior whose purpose is usually to provide sensory stimulation) while playing, are they able to independently get back on task and finish the activity?
- If I set my child up in a room with minimal distractions and the items needed to complete the activity, can they stay engaged in the activity for at least five minutes without my involvement (I am in the room, but I'm not guiding them back to the area, encouraging them to continue playing, or talking to them)?

Engagement in Nonpreferred Activities

DESCRIPTION: The ability to stay on task and complete a single, nonpreferred activity (for example homework, picking up toys, or taking a shower) with an adult present.

SCENARIOS:

1. Your child does not love to sit at the table and eat. If left to themselves, they would wander around the house with their food. However, if you are sitting at the table with them, they will remain seated with no problem behaviors and eat their food at the table.
2. Your child does not love working with their therapist. They would not spontaneously request to do therapy activities if the therapist was not there. However, they will independently remain in an assigned area and willingly work with the therapist during sessions.

WHY IT'S IMPORTANT: Using a task analysis to teach daily living skills will probably require your child to complete activities they'd likely prefer not to complete. That's why your child's ability to remain in one area and perform a single, nonpreferred task, with an adult present, is a prerequisite for this program.

QUESTIONS TO ASK YOURSELF:

- If I present my child with an open-ended, nonpreferred activity (building with blocks or pretend play), will they stay engaged in the activity for five minutes with adult engagement?
- If I present my child with a closed-ended, nonpreferred activity (picking up

toys or putting on their jacket) and stay in the area, will my child stay on task until the activity is completed?
- If my child receives therapy of any kind, do they willingly participate in sessions?

Following Directions in Context

DESCRIPTION: The ability to follow directions for a nonpreferred activity within the environment that the activity is taking place.

SCENARIOS:

1. You ask your child to wash their hands after going to the bathroom because handwashing naturally follows using the bathroom, you are still in the bathroom, and they can follow the sequence to some degree. In this case, whether your child can follow through completely on the directive isn't important. What's important is that they attempt to complete the first step, letting you know that they understood the direction. For example, they may not be washing their hands thoroughly or know how to get the soap, but if you say, "Let's wash your hands," they will walk to the sink and at least attempt to turn on the water or place their hands under the faucet.
2. You ask your child to put their plate in the sink following dinner because cleaning up naturally occurs after eating dinner, and you are still in the kitchen. They pick up their plate and walk toward the sink. Again, completing what you ask isn't the skill; it's that they make an effort to do so.

WHY IT'S IMPORTANT: For your child to make progress in this program, we want to make sure that they have some understanding of simple routines, a basic ability to follow directions in context, and the willingness to complete nonpreferred tasks when asked to do so. This skill relies on visual and situational prompts embedded in the environment, which you'll learn more about in Chapter 4, so it's important to assess whether your child can follow this type of direction.

QUESTIONS TO ASK YOURSELF:
- If you give your child a direction within the context of an everyday routine, will they follow the direction? Examples include the direction to put their

clothes in the hamper when changing into their pajamas, to put on their coat when leaving for school, or to get their cup when they ask you for more water.

Following a Cue versus Following a Directive

Sometimes children do something not because there was a verbal directive, but because they have paired that behavior with another cue in the environment. For example, a parent is ready to go out and says, "Get your shoes" to her child. The child comes running to her with his shoes. She thinks he is following the direction. In actuality, the child saw her get her car keys and automatically ran over to get his shoes because he loves going in the car. This skill generally comes before following directions. If your child can do this, great! However, it does not count as following directions. You want to make sure your child is capable of engaging in an activity because he understands what was asked of him.

Ability to Accept Prompts

DESCRIPTION: When unable to complete a task independently, your child allows you to physically assist them (called a *physical prompt*) or can follow a *visual cue* to get the job done.

SCENARIOS:

1. Your child is having trouble cutting their food with a knife, but allows you to put your hand over their hand to show them how.
2. Your child is putting away their toys but is unsure where a toy goes. They see you point to the bin that it goes in and follow your direction to put the toy in that bin.

WHY IT'S IMPORTANT: Having this skill means that your child knows how to learn—that they can accept physical prompting or follow visual cues when needed to complete a task.

QUESTIONS TO ASK YOURSELF:

- Does your child look to you for direction and guidance?
- Does your child accept physical prompts or follow visual prompts like pointing or a visual schedule when they are offered?
- Does your child follow adult directives?

Ability to Accept Redirection

DESCRIPTION: A technique used to direct a child from engaging in a problem behavior to a more appropriate behavior.

SCENARIOS:

1. Your child is in the process of brushing their teeth. In the middle of the sequence, he stops to play with the water. You direct him back to brushing his teeth by pointing to the handle of the toothbrush, and he picks up the toothbrush.
2. You ask your child to clean up their toys. In the process of cleaning up their toys, they start playing with their iPad. You redirect them back to cleaning up their toys by saying, "It's not time for your iPad. Please finish cleaning up," and they finish cleaning up.

WHY IT'S IMPORTANT: Getting off task happens to all of us. The key, though, is the ability to refocus once redirected. Your child must be able to accept redirection in a simple situation without engaging in tantrum behavior, self-injurious behavior, or any other problem behavior.

QUESTIONS TO ASK YOURSELF:

- If your child is not doing what they need to be doing, and you attempt to guide them back to the task (either physically, verbally, or visually), are they able to accept this redirection and get back on task without engaging in problem behavior?

Stereotypic Behavior

Within the topic of redirection, there are two subtopics we would like to mention: repetitive movements and restricted interests. It is okay if your child engages in these behaviors if they are safe and able to stay on task or are redirectable back to task with minimal involvement from others.

Repetitive Movements

DESCRIPTION: A repetitive behavior whose purpose is usually to provide sensory stimulation such as hand flapping, jumping, eye gazing (holding items close to their eyes and staring at them for an extended amount of time), or making repetitive sounds. Please note that the aforementioned are considered safe stereotypic behaviors; unsafe stereotypic behaviors such as head banging, pulling out hair, or picking at skin are not safe and are addressed in the "Self-injurious behavior" section earlier in this chapter.

SCENARIOS:

1. Your child is completing a puzzle, stops in the middle to hand flap for five seconds, and then independently goes back to completing the puzzle.
2. Your child is brushing their teeth and stops in the middle to hum loudly, but resumes brushing their teeth when you point to the toothbrush.

QUESTIONS TO ASK YOURSELF:

- Is my child able to independently get back on task if they stop to engage in stereotypic behavior during a task?
- Am I able to redirect my child back to a task if they are engaged in a stereotypic behavior?

Restrictive Interests

DESCRIPTION: These include behaviors such as hyperfixation, adhering to rituals, and rigid focus on a narrow range of topics. Many times, children with ASD engage in repetitive and restricted behaviors, such as an adherence to routine. These behaviors are sometimes referred to as OCD-like behaviors, but do not warrant having a separate diagnosis of OCD (obsessive–compulsive disorder).

SCENARIOS:

1. You need to stop at the store on the way home from picking your child up at school. You never do this, and your child has a tantrum because you strayed from your usual routine.

2. You decide to rearrange the furniture in the living room to accommodate a new armchair you purchased. Your child is distraught that you rearranged the furniture and put something new in the room.
3. Your child wants to tell you about dinosaurs, recite the presidents, discuss the train schedule, or converse about some other topic of interest to them. You have asked them to eat their lunch, but they will not move on until they have finished telling you every last detail they want to tell you.
4. Your child wants you to play princess figurines with her, but she only wants you to play the exact way she wants. Your child needs the princess to go up to the tower and then fall into a pit while she sings a specific song, and she will become upset if the script cannot be completed. This is an example of a repetitive or stereotypic behavior. Although play routines can be appropriate, they are a problem when they become overly rigid and your child refuses to modify them or incorporate other suggestions for how to play.

QUESTIONS TO ASK YOURSELF:

- Is my child able to get back on task if they are distracted by a repetitive movement or restricted interest in the middle of completing the task?
- Am I able to redirect my child if they are engaged in one of their nonfunctional, self-made routines (routines that they created for the sole purpose of bringing them sensory stimulation or relief)?

Ability to Understand the "First, Then" Concept

DESCRIPTION: The ability to engage in a nonpreferred task *first*, with the understanding that you will *then* be able to engage in a preferred task upon its completion. In behavioral terms, this is known as the Premack principle. In layman's terms, it is affectionately called "Grandma's rule." The idea is, first you eat your broccoli, then you can have a cookie.

SCENARIOS:

1. You tell your child that they can watch television after their therapy session, and they actively participate in therapy before turning on the television.
2. You tell your child that they can play outside after they pick up the craft supplies they were using, and they calmly clean up before going outside.

WHY IT'S IMPORTANT: Your child should be able to delay engagement in a preferred activity until after they have completed a nonpreferred activity. This goes back to the concept of self-direction and the ability to eventually initiate tasks they don't want to do even when they have access to activities they'd rather be doing.

QUESTIONS TO ASK YOURSELF:

- Does my child understand and tolerate "first this, then that"? This can be presented either verbally or visually.

ACTIVITY: Foundational Learning Skills Assessment

Now let's determine which foundational learning skills your child has by completing the following assessment. Please remember to score based on situations when your child is being asked to do nonpreferred tasks, has the freedom to leave the designated area, and is not bribed, coaxed, or promised a highly preferred item or activity. You can be present during the activity, but your child should not require prompting other than to get started.

Skill	YES, my child does have this skill	NO, my child does not have this skill
Able to stay engaged in preferred activities for at least 5 minutes		
Able to stay engaged in nonpreferred activities for at least 5 minutes		
Follows directions in context		
Accepts prompts		
Accepts redirection		
Understands "first, then" concept		

HELP! MY CHILD CAN'T DO SOME OR ALL OF THESE SKILLS: The foundational skills listed in this chapter are the basis for everything else you will teach your child. The more proficient your child is in these skills early on, the easier it will be to teach higher-level skills later. These skills take time to learn, though, and not all children will learn them naturally as they go through life without direct teaching. If your child can learn them in the natural environment without instruction, great. If they cannot—and many children with learning differences are not able to learn that way—these skills are best taught using a structured and systematic approach. Many times, children who struggle to learn in a typical environment thrive in a structured learning environment. Structured learning environments provide opportunities for repetition and consistent reinforcement following correct responding. As with the unsafe behaviors, you may find that you can teach your child the foundational skills needed by referencing books or other online resources, or you may find you need to seek the help of a professional.

This chapter should have given you a good idea about whether or not your child has the safety behaviors and skills needed to be successful with this program. If they are engaging in unsafe behavior, your next step is to secure the appropriate guidance needed to help you teach your child appropriate replacement behaviors. If they are lacking in any of the needed skills, seek out any additional help you may need to teach them those skills before moving on with this program. If they can be trusted to be safe *and* are proficient in the skills presented here—fantastic! They are ready to increase their independence. However, you don't have the all-clear yet to move forward, as we haven't discussed the other part of this team—you! In the next chapter, you'll be invited to assess your readiness to start implementing the strategies presented later in the book. These two chapters—the one you just read and the one you are about to read—are important to creating a solid foundation to maximize your ability to teach and your child's ability to learn. Let's check back in with Lisa and her three children.

Who Is Ready?

Lisa decided it was time to start teaching her kids how to be more independent. After reading Chapter 3 of *Spectrum of Independence: How to Teach Your Neurodiverse Child Daily Life Skills,* she realized that not all of her children were ready. Her son Chris was definitely ready—he did not have any unsafe behaviors and had all of the prerequisite skills needed to be successful with the program. Her son Jack had some unsafe behaviors that she would need to address before she could really start the program with him. Although she would be able to teach him some skills, like hanging up his coat, and modify the environment to help him be successful, she would not be able to carry out the fading steps and remove herself from the routine until she addressed his elopement and pica. Laura was really close to being ready. She did not have any unsafe behaviors and had most of the prerequisite skills. Laura needed to practice completing nonpreferred tasks without so much redirection. Lisa would ask Laura's classroom teacher to practice those skills with her to help get her ready to be more independent too.

4

"Are You Ready for This?"
EVALUATING YOUR OWN READINESS

Madeline took a deep breath and counted to five. Her cellphone had pinged with email, text, and calendar notifications almost continuously while she tried to get her daughter, Addie, settled in after school. Addie got off the bus talking about how she wanted an Elsa backpack to match her favorite Elsa toy. Madeline tried to get her to talk about how her school day went and other social questions, but Addie kept coming back to Elsa. Madeline felt her anxiety spike as her phone rang. Was it the plumber or electrician? She was trying to manage what was supposed to be a small bathroom remodel, but it was turning into a full-scale project. She looked at Addie and said, "Take out your folder, put your backpack away, and go sit at the kitchen table," before moving to pick up her phone. She tried not to think about how few of those instructions her daughter was likely to follow. In the back of her mind, Madeline wondered if Addie would ever be able to do things by herself.

"Oh," she thought. It wasn't about the remodel. The school was calling . . . again. Madeline almost let out a muttered curse but stopped herself just in time. Addie was an excellent mimic when it came to four-letter words. Madeline's mind raced. Was this about the IEP meeting next week, just a check-in, or bad news about Addie's behavior? The list of possibilities was endless. Madeline sighed and answered. She quickly realized it was just an automated message telling her that Addie had been tardy to class, which she hadn't because she was in a self-contained classroom that didn't change classes during the day. Annoying.

Adding the return call she'd need to make to her ever-growing mental list of Things to Deal with Later, she turned around. Addie had wandered over to the kitchen table, still telling Madeline excitedly about the Elsa backpack. Frozen was her current favorite thing. Madeline sighed again. She debated asking Addie to do the tasks once more and changed her mind. She didn't have the energy or the time. Instead, she got some carrot sticks out of the fridge and put them on the table. She looked over. Addie had found the iPad on the chair in the kitchen that Madeline had meant to put away this morning. This time, Madeline did curse, but very quietly. She knew that once Addie started a YouTube video, getting her back on track was a losing battle. She took the backpack off her daughter's back, got out the folder, and repeated herself (for what felt like the millionth time today), "Sit in the chair and eat your carrots," while pointing. Addie continued to play with the iPad and hum.

Madeline knew that her frustration wasn't her daughter's fault. In addition to her 9-year-old daughter with autism, Madeline had 15-year-old twin boys and a toddler. She thought to herself, "I'm just tired. I am a good mom, and I am doing my best." She breathed slowly in and out to a count of five until her heartbeat returned to normal. As she sat down to look at Addie's folder, she wished her husband didn't have to travel for work. But he did. She wished that her parents lived closer than two hours away and didn't pressure her to visit them instead of coming to help, but that felt impossible to ask for. She wished Addie's behavior therapists offered in-home therapy, but they didn't. She wished she had friends who could come over, but her friends were busy too. She wished that she hadn't been up last night worrying about her daughter's future, but of course she had been, as she often was. She wished she wasn't so overwhelmed and desperate for more time and energy to spend helping her daughter, but she didn't know where to start.

You may be familiar with the phrase "Put your own oxygen mask on first before you help others." This isn't just a rule from the airlines. It's a valuable metaphor for how to prepare for behavior change—your own and your child's. Yes, the strategies in our book can help with some aspects of stress, particularly related to your child's ability to be independent, but the strategies work best if the appropriate supports *for you* are in place first. This chapter will help you determine whether you are ready to implement this program and give you some ideas for how to decrease some of the barriers that may hinder your success.

As educators, we would never expect a child to succeed without the right supports. Yet for some reason, our culture has different expectations for adults. We treat adults like they can operate in isolation and are somehow totally in control of their environment and the events around them. Surprise! They aren't. Parents can't control many things, including the attitudes of family and friends, the services a given therapist offers, the robocalls from the school, and even your child's insistence that TV shows about dinosaurs are the best. However, there are decisions that parents can make that set them and their child up for success. If the environment is supportive, success is much more likely. The question is, how much are you willing *and* able to change about your own life?

Evaluating Your Circumstances

Let's take stock of the potential barriers to starting and maintaining the behavior change needed to see improvements in your child's independence. What is your stress level like? What is going on daily, or what is on the horizon, that might keep you from being able to dedicate time and consistency to teaching your child independent task management? Let's find out.

- **Major life events:** Have you had any major life events recently that are still affecting you? Here are some examples, but any out-of-the-ordinary, stressful event would fall into this category.
  - Death in the family or close support network
  - Birth in the family
  - Illness in the family or close support network (long term, requiring increased care, or causing increased stress)
  - Move to a new home
  - Construction on current home
  - Transfer or graduation from school for the child with a disability
  - Family member or support person experiencing a major surgery or extended hospital stay; this could be for either physical or mental health reasons
- **Logistics:** Do you have any changes to your regular routine coming up in the near future?
  - Long vacations and summer holidays
  - School breaks or school starting again
  - Starting or terminating therapy, after-school program, or new daycare

- Extended family visiting or staying in your home
- Extended visit to family

- **Time commitment:** Do you have 30 minutes a day for the next three to six weeks to commit to one of your child's routines (toothbrushing, getting dressed, showering)?

- **Increasing your consistency:** Are you willing to become a consistent and predictable source of both reinforcement and boundaries for your child? Are you prepared to stick to your word?

- **Emotional considerations:** Do you have three to five stress-reduction or coping techniques you use regularly with success?

- **A Supportive environment:** Is your home free from distractions that your child finds irresistible (probably electronics, if we had to guess)? Or does it contain disturbances, such as TVs on in the background, phone and alarm dings, or barking dogs that might impede learning? Can your child reach and find all the things they need?

- **Believing:** Do you believe your child is capable of learning to be more independent?

- **Your support network:** Do you have anyone you feel safe leaving your child with? For how long? Under what circumstances? Does your child work with any therapists? Are you willing to ask them for support?

Please complete the Assessing for Barriers form on page 78.

How did you fare? If you're like most of the parents we work with, you might be feeling worried about a few areas. That's okay! None of us have perfect lives, and we certainly don't believe you need to have one to make the strategies in this book work for you and your child. However, we can all probably make small changes in one or more areas so that we set ourselves up for success. Oxygen for you *first*, remember? That said, if after reading this section you feel that too many barriers are stacked up against you, and progress won't be possible at this time, please continue to read this chapter. The rest of this chapter will give you some ideas for how you can begin the process of addressing those barriers. We hope this will help you build stability and support in your home so you can begin working with your child to increase their independence.

Major Life Events

If you answered "yes" to any of the major life events noted on page 63, particularly if they have thrown off your family's routine or way of living your daily life, we suggest waiting to start this book until your life has settled back into a routine. Due to the time and energy that these activities will require of you, it is best to be in a settled routine before starting. Additionally, the data may not be consistent until a routine is established. Just like your own behavior may be affected by a major life event, there will be increased variability, increased frustrations, and increased disruptions in your child's life as well. That is totally normal, but as you'll learn (or have already learned), we are focused on setting everyone in your child's life (parents, therapist, child, siblings, and other family members) up for success. This will look different for each person, but any of these examples of life upheavals will set you up for increased frustration and failure that are not the fault of you or your child.

Logistics

If your schedule is inconsistent due to outside circumstances, this will make being consistent for your child much more difficult. While variety is the spice of life, for most people, a routine can provide stability, predictability, and consistency. These are particularly important for children with autism and anxiety. If you are planning a big event in the near future or are just coming back from one (trip, family visit, school break), it would be best to give your schedule time to stabilize before beginning the activities in this book. This will also help with accurate data collection. Think about yourself. When you aren't at your best because you are anxious, tired, or stressed, you are probably not going to perform at your best either. Therefore, if your child is tired and overwhelmed, it's okay to wait a bit until things settle down. Additionally, if you're about to go on vacation where you know you won't be able to do the routine, it's probably not the best time to start either. We want the data to be taken when your child is at their best and when the routine can be completed consistently.

You know your child best. You will know when things have become more routine. We leave this up to your judgment but want you to be cautious. While we know our book will just be so inspirational and you'll want to get right up and start today (please interpret this with sarcasm), we want you to be fully prepared before committing to completing the activities. It's for your sake and your child's.

Time Commitment

First, if you're already reading this book, we appreciate your time. Now (and throughout this book), we're going to ask for more. We're going to ask you to record your child while they complete routines like getting ready in the morning, or in the afternoon while they do their after-school routine. We're going to ask you to watch those videos and document what types of support you are giving your child throughout the process, like verbally telling your child to brush their teeth, pointing to the toothbrush, or physically helping them to grasp the toothbrush. For example, we know that Madeline gave verbal (spoken) and gestural (pointing at or motioning toward) prompts that Addie didn't respond to, and then did the tasks for Addie when the prompts didn't work. Taking these data will take time. Time you might feel like you don't have. We challenge you to think about the long game.

While this initial investment in your child's independence will ask for extra effort and time on your part, let's consider how much time those daily routines take right now. You could start by simply timing how long it takes you to get your child ready for school each morning or to get your child ready for bed each night. Now imagine getting some (or all) of that time back to do with as you please. For Madeline, that might mean extra time to talk with friends on the phone, extra energy for her other children, or simply an additional 20 minutes in her day to drink hot coffee instead of cold coffee out of the microwave (once she could remember where she put it . . .).

Also, consider how you could get some time back to complete the activities in this book. This may mean delegating some of your home responsibilities to a spouse or family member, hiring someone to do some home tasks, or temporarily refocusing your priorities so that you can eliminate certain tasks from your schedule. Once you have committed to devoting time to teaching your child independent living skills, it may be easier to set boundaries around your time and say no to things that are unnecessarily sapping you of energy, like manning the table at the school bake sale or attending a social function that you don't want to go to.

Increasing Your Consistency

It can be very tempting to abandon consistency when the everyday stressors of getting the kids in bed on time start to weigh on you. We know the classic dinner dilemma. You're in the middle of stirring the spaghetti sauce and you can't step away from the stove. You've just said it's time to sit down for dinner, and your child is still in the living room playing with toys. You can either ignore them ignoring you and bring them their dinner in the living room, which is easier in the moment, or walk into the living room and risk burning the sauce. Taking the time to walk over, show your child that the timer is going off, and help them get to the table is the harder choice because they might whine or even resort to a full-blown tantrum. Lots of factors play into consistency. Your level of stress, what's going on around you, your child's past reactions to your attempts at consistency, and even the time of day make it easier or harder to be consistent. We are asking you to commit to consistency as you are working on the skills they need to care for themselves on a daily basis. We will discuss this further in Chapter 5, but here's a sneak peek. Consistency is what makes behavioral interventions effective. Without it, you're setting you and your child up for a longer, more challenging journey to independence.

Emotional Considerations

In the next chapter, we will ask you to assess your emotional readiness to be consistent with your directives. Can you stay calm when your child is upset or frustrated? What strategies did Madeline use when she was feeling stressed and anxious? If you don't remember, go back to the vignette. Were the strategies successful? Why or why not?

Do you have successful coping strategies that you use? If not, would you be willing to find ones that work for you? We recommend having a set of effective coping strategies and using them in your daily routines for at least a few weeks before beginning the teaching portion of this book. If you struggle to regulate your own emotions and model appropriate coping skills for your child, this process may be very difficult.

Again, we're back to the long game. Yes, initially, any behavior change can be stressful. Even taking a different or unknown route to work can feel stressful in the moment. However, think about the long-term impact of decreasing your stress around daily routines for your child, as well as worries about their health and safety as they grow into adolescents and adults. We believe that a small initial increase in time commitment and stress are worth it in the long run. But this isn't our time and our stress, it's yours. And the decision to undertake and stick to what we are asking you to do is also up to you. Each day, possibly multiple times a day, you may be tempted to give in, abandon your plan and strategies, and just do the task for your child. However, these choices only guarantee one thing—everything will stay the same. Your child will not magically develop these skills. You will very likely continue to help them complete the same routines each day exactly as you are now unless something changes. What we are asking you to do may be uncomfortable, but temporary discomfort can result in a future increase in your freedom as well as your child's. We believe it is worth it, and hopefully you do too.

A Supportive Environment

At different points in the book, we will ask you to assess your home environment for barriers and fix those problems. If your child is easily distracted by toys or electronics, we may ask you to remove them temporarily from where the instruction is taking place. Places such as the bedroom, bathroom, kitchen, entryway, or mudroom are common places for daily routines to take place. We may also ask you to hold electronics access until morning and afternoon routines are complete. We also ask you to assess how your child completes a routine and structural issues that may arise. We may ask you to replace a squeeze tube of toothpaste with an automatic toothpaste dispenser or a bar of soap with a child-friendly soap dispenser. To assist with the afternoon routine, are you willing to purchase prepackaged snacks or are you willing to prepackage snacks yourself so your child can access them independently? If getting dressed is hard because your child wants to wear the same shirt over and over again, are you willing to buy five shirts with characters on them so they can wear one each day, to increase their motivation to get dressed and decrease problem behavior in the mornings?

Did any of these scenarios give you pause? Did you feel any resistance to those ideas and changes? Why is that? Is it a logistical barrier or an emotional one? Logistical barriers are relatively easy to overcome with some creativity, but emotional barriers may require more consideration. Think about why this makes you, as the parent, feel anxious, upset, or uncomfortable. While many people experience anxiety, if it is impacting your ability to help your child move forward, we recommend trying some new strategies to address your feelings. As we said earlier, figuring out how to regulate your own reactions will help you and your child be successful. If you are feeling anxious about changes, you may want to get assistance from a therapist or counselor. If that is cost-prohibitive or not available to you for other reasons, you may find online resources including apps for anxiety and stress helpful. Making lists of what is causing your anxiety, and then checking back on that a week later to see what has resolved may also be a good practice to add to your routine. This can help you determine which stressors are resolved with time, and which need continued action to resolve.

When assessing Madeline and Addie's environment, the first thing that comes to mind are some logistical questions. Does Addie know where her backpack goes? Does she have a designated hook that is always available for her to hang up her backpack? Does she know which folder to get out of her backpack? Would she have been more likely to follow directions if they were broken down into individual directions instead of given three at a time? What if the iPad was put away and not a distraction? There are many ways to modify the environment to set your child up for success. We will ask you to assess the environment (your home) to see if there are any opportunities for decluttering, clearing, and simplifying.

Believing Your Child Is Capable

Your beliefs about your child also impact your ability to stick to a plan and see it through. Do you believe that your child can learn? Madeline worries that Addie will never learn to do the activities of daily living independently. While it's okay and very normal to have these worries, we ask for you to remain hopeful and to set high expectations for your child. Since you are reading this book, we are hopeful that you do believe in the potential for your child to be independent. If you do not believe in that possibility, we'd like you to examine that belief. Where does it come from? It might come from many years of trying to help your child and not seeing results. Or it may come from the opinions of people you trust, such as educators and experts, who have spent years telling you (either outright or in their actions) that your child will never attain certain goals. Either way, consider this: Trying a new technique holds the potential for a different—a better—outcome.

The best way to stay where you are is to keep doing what you are doing right now. We are asking you to try something different and keep an open mind about the possible outcomes your child may attain. We know that these strategies can work because they are scientifically based, and we have seen our students' and clients' progress over time. We are asking you to place your trust in the science, in yourself, and in your child.

Building Your Support Network

Many parents with neurodiverse children feel completely alone. However, most people have some supports, and those resources may be untapped. This could include your spiritual or church community, immediate and extended family, school support personnel, online support groups, therapists, neighbors, members of your cultural community, fellow parents, friends, and your spouse or partner. One of the benefits of community building is that you may ask for and receive support from people outside of your direct family members. You may also have some or all of the following specialists and professionals assisting with your child: behavior analyst, registered behavior technician, occupational therapist, speech therapist or speech language pathologist, physical therapist, and medical providers.

Many people have been taught that individualism is king and that to admit you need help is weakness or defeat. And sure, it is important to be able to handle some things by yourself, but it can be beneficial to raise your children in the context of a larger community and family support. This allows you to take a break sometimes and seek support more easily. Although we realize this can be challenging to accomplish, by thinking outside the box, oftentimes these communities can be built.

The first step to getting help is admitting that you need it. It sounds simple, but this can take deep mental work. That is totally okay. The second step is to think of what tasks you need help with. Then you need to find a person in your community who can help. Be sure to match the task to the abilities of the person. Then you have to actually ask for the help. Be specific and direct, and you may want to explain why or for how long the help will be needed. Depending on your culture, you may want to offer to pay or to trade for this help. One option is to trade babysitting with another family so that couples can switch off having a date night.

As an extra wrinkle in the process of asking for help, remember that not all help is created equal. You may enjoy some free time because your sister is babysitting, but you may also come home to a messy kitchen and a child who had gummy bears and ice cream for dinner. We're giving a silly example, but the effects of inconsistency in schedules, consequences, and how an adult reacts to situations can have a significant impact on child behavior. Children with disabilities are very capable of learning that there are different rules with different people. However, this is an extra and unnecessary hurdle to independence, particularly at the beginning of this independence journey. This may also cause problem behavior; for example, Grandma doesn't make me brush my teeth, so when Dad asks me to, I'm upset. Either way, we want to stack the deck in favor of your child's success, not throw up extra barriers from other adults.

The additional support from your community may also come with some challenges, particularly if you were raised in a family that is wary of outside help. There is no simple solution to these issues. Family dynamics are complicated and very culturally dependent. You may need to have an honest conversation with yourself about what's best for your child and their future. You may need to break family tradition, and are you ready for what that might mean? Perhaps feelings will be bruised initially, but over time the progress you and your child make will hopefully be the evidence that you made the right decision.

How to Assess Your Situation

Let's go back to Madeline and her daughter Addie. How prepared is Madeline to take on the tasks of this book with her current circumstances? Are there things within her control that she could do to make any behavioral changes more likely to succeed? What could those changes be?

At the end of this chapter, you'll complete two additional worksheets: Classifying Stressors and Brainstorming Solutions. For now, let's look at how Madeline would have filled them out, on the upcoming pages.

Example of Assessing for Barriers

Potential stressors	This is a concern	This is not a concern
Major life events: We have had a major life event recently that is still affecting me, my child, or other family members.	✓—renovation	
Logistics: We will have changes to our regular routine coming up in the near future.		✓
Time commitment: I have 30 minutes a day for the next 3–6 weeks to commit to one of my child's routines (e.g., toothbrushing).	✓—Too much to do, can't imagine giving up 30 minutes a day	
Increasing your consistency: I am willing to become a consistent and predictable source of both reinforcement and boundaries for my child. I am prepared to stick to my word.	✓—I know I need to stick to my word, but I'm pretty overwhelmed	
Emotional considerations: I have 3–5 stress-reduction or coping techniques that I use regularly with success.	✓—Again, just stressed to the max. I know I can count to 10 and breathe, but that doesn't always work	
A supportive environment: My home is free from distractions so that my child can focus. My child can reach and find all the things they need.	✓—Nope, iPad is out, sometimes the TV is on, and my kids are noisy	
Believing: I believe my child is capable of learning to be more independent.	✓—I do, secretly, worry about this	
Your support network: I have people that I feel safe leaving my child with. My child works with specialists.	✓—Her grandparents, but they're far away. She does have a behavior analyst, but they don't do in-home training or services	

Now let's see how Madeline classified her stressors.

Example of Classifying Stressors

Completely within my control	Somewhat within my control	Completely out of my control
Increasing consistency—it's hard to stay consistent when I tell Addie to do things, I'm usually tired and think it's easier to just do it for her	Bathroom remodel	Support network: Husband's work schedule Parents live 2 hours away
Emotional considerations—I have some stress-reduction techniques, but I probably need more	Time commitment—I can't tell if this is real or if I'm just so stressed that it doesn't feel like I have that extra time	School phone calls
Believing in Addie	Support network—no social time with friends	ABA services not available at home
Supportive environment—picking up electronics and toys	Big worries about Addie's future	
Phone notifications		

On to the good stuff, the solutions! Madeline probably had to work on this list over time (see the worksheet on page 77). We don't expect you to have all the answers in an initial read-through of this book. But we do want to challenge you to not skip over anything. Just like Madeline did, it's okay to say that something feels hard right now and that you'll come back to it. Acknowledging the problem may lead you to think about it in a new way, discuss it with others, and get creative.

How does Madeline's experience match up with yours? How is it different? Are there things that Madeline is dealing with that you can empathize with? Let's take that forward and see how Madeline decided to go about making time to do the extra work that this book is asking for.

Fast-Forward: Madeline Makes Changes

Next we present a few of the ways that Madeline changed her environment to increase her own readiness. We know each family has different circumstances, but we hope you can take some inspiration from this vignette and look at your life with a new and more critical eye. What are your stressors, and how can you address them so you can be more present and available to help build your child's independence?

> It had taken four months, but Madeline had done it. She knew she needed to change, but looking at the whole picture was overwhelming, so she started with the annoying stuff. She began placing her phone to "Do not disturb" once she got home from work. The settings allowed her preferred contacts to ring through, but everything else was silent. Yes, the bathroom remodel was small and didn't throw off their daily routine, but it was taking up lots of her valuable mental space. She'd decided to put her husband in charge of those calls. He could answer even when he was traveling for work, so she'd delegated those responsibilities to him. She also selected a specific ringtone for the school, and as long as Addie was with her, she didn't answer because she knew it wasn't an emergency. She'd listen to the messages once things weren't hectic and send an email response so she wasn't playing phone tag with the attendance office or the teacher.
>
> Next, she turned her attention to recruiting more help. She had very serious sit-down discussions with her parents and her 15-year-old twins. For her parents, she'd calmly told them that their constant invitations to visit were not, in fact, helpful at all, but placed extra pressure on her to coordinate and plan travel. She explained that the twins had practices and school events, that their house wasn't toddler-proof, and that taking four hours of driving plus the visit time out of her already packed schedule was nearly impossible. She told her parents what would actually help: if one of them came to stay with her when her husband was out of town to help with the kids. Her parents, both retired and unaware of Madeline's specific struggles, agreed to switch off which one of them would visit for one week out of the month while her husband was gone.

To her twins, she'd decreed that they would be responsible for dinner (including adding the ingredients to the shared family grocery list phone app) two nights a week. One would cook, the other would do the dishes, and then they'd switch for the second night. She only had one rule: They had to have at least a vegetable side dish. Yes, she now ate more meals of premade ravioli and frozen pizza and a "salad," but she was willing to sacrifice her taste buds for the freedom from cooking and washing dishes. And her toddler was ecstatic about the new chefs' culinary decisions. She also contacted the twins' friends' parents to ask if they could start a carpool to some of the (very many) practices for sports, theater, and band. Those parents were relieved to split the drives with her. Now she was only driving to 5 different places a week instead of 15.

Once she freed up some time, she felt more open (and less guilty) about doing things for herself. She started seeing a therapist to learn coping strategies for feelings of stress, overwhelm, frustration, and annoyance. The therapist provided remote services, so Madeline sat in her car once a week at lunch for her sessions. At her therapist's urging, she also scheduled a once-a-month standing hangout with friends. It's casual and people come and go based on their availability, but it allows Madeline to get out of the house and have social time for herself. Madeline also started using a mindfulness app to practice keeping her cool in stressful situations both at home and work. Madeline contacted a financial planner and had an initial meeting with her. The financial planner explained to Madeline that there were ways to set up trusts to provide for Addie's care if something were to happen to Madeline and her husband. They also discussed setting up a savings account for Addie to be used toward an inclusive higher education program after she completes high school. Madeline scheduled meetings with other family members and the financial planner to iron out details for Addie's future and finances. While this didn't completely erase Madeline's fears, she found that she had an easier time falling asleep.

Then, feeling more fulfilled, rested, and supported, she started to look around for resources to help Addie. She posted in a local autism parent group and asked which service providers offered in-home therapy. She got some names and put Addie on waiting lists. She also talked to their current provider about her concerns about Addie's independence. The behavior analyst was responsive and provided feedback on what Madeline decided to do at home.

Madeline added a picture of Addie's folder to the place on the kitchen table where she wanted Addie to put it and showed Addie how to put her folder there. Madeline also hung a hook at Addie's height at the door from the garage with her daughter's name over it. She took a picture of Addie's backpack as it hung on the wall and printed and hung it underneath the hook as a visual example. She, her husband, or one of her parents made sure the kitchen was clear of toys and electronics before Addie came home. Madeline used the time after school to work with Addie on being independent, eventually progressing to having Addie put her shoes away, change out of her school clothes and into comfortable clothes laid out on her bed, wash her hands, and sit down at the counter to eat her snack.

In our example, Madeline started with the small, annoying, and easily solvable pieces of her situation. Once those were addressed, Madeline began to tap into something called *behavioral momentum*. This is the concept that once we have small successes that result in reinforcement, we are more likely to attempt and complete harder behaviors and tasks. Also, lowering her overall stress level across the day freed up some mental space for Madeline to consider her larger and more difficult-to-solve pieces of the puzzle. Some people might do this in the reverse order (most difficult to least) or work on various problems simultaneously. There is no right or wrong way to go about addressing these problems.

Your preferences, your particular situation, the time available for these activities, and your specific barriers should all be considered. We provided you an example of each worksheet filled out from Madeline's perspective to use for inspiration. We suggest completing these worksheets for yourself, then prioritizing which issue to begin with first. As one issue is solved or causes less stress, you can turn your attention to another area. This process may take a significant amount of time, and that is fine. We encourage you to address the issues with a consistent focus until you feel ready to address your child's independent living skills. Time to get started taking those barriers on!

Let's move on to the worksheet Brainstorming Solutions. Notice that some things were totally overwhelming for Madeline, so she had to handle other things first. She's being brutally honest in her responses, and we hope you do the same. This book is for you, so now is the time to be clear with yourself about the availability of solutions to your problems. Please feel free to gather information from the people around you too. There may be people in your life with suggestions about what can help or who are willing to contribute to your efforts. Feel free to return to this worksheet and add your new ideas or any new problems you have noticed.

Example of Brainstorming Solutions

Problem	Solution
Bathroom remodel	Delegate to my husband
Parents live 2 hours away	Ask them to come help or at least ask them to stop asking for visits because that stresses me out
Time commitment	Have the twins make dinner twice a week or even do those pickup meals
Supportive environment—picking up electronics and toys	I think I can do a sweep before she gets home and her dad can do one on the days I can't. We just need to communicate about it.
Increasing consistency—it's hard to stay consistent when I tell Addie to do things, I'm usually tired and think it's easier to just do it for her	I'm not sure what to do about this. Maybe once I get the other things out of the way, this will be easier?
Believing in Addie	This feels really hard right now. Hopefully once I see some progress this will get easier.
Emotional considerations—I have some stress-reduction techniques, but I probably need more	I probably need to start therapy and get one of those mindfulness apps I've seen ads for.
Phone notifications	I've been meaning to set up those "focus modes" on my phone so only certain notifications from certain people come through. I'll do that for work and school notifications.
Support network—no social time with friends	I miss my friends. I feel hopeful that once I get things together, I can see them more. Maybe a monthly trip to our favorite Mexican restaurant?
ABA services not available at home	I can put Addie on waitlists for other providers who do have in-home services.
Big worries about Addie's future	I should probably figure out who to talk to about this. Financial planner? Lawyer? Both? It feels overwhelming to even think about that.

Once you have finished with the problem-solving worksheets, (hopefully!) most of the barriers to success have been at least partially addressed. Now comes the time to decide if you're ready to move forward. Do you feel you can devote 30 minutes to this every day for the next three to six weeks? Do you feel supported enough to do so? If so, welcome to Part III of this book.

Assessing for Barriers

Place a checkmark in the appropriate box for each potential stressor.

Potential stressors	This is a concern	This is not a concern
Major life events: We have had a major life event recently that is still affecting me, my child, or other family members.		
Logistics: We will have changes to our regular routine coming up in the near future.		
Time commitment: I have 30 minutes a day for the next 3–6 weeks to commit to one of my child's routines (e.g., toothbrushing).		
Increasing your consistency: I am willing to become a consistent and predictable source of both reinforcement and boundaries for my child. I am prepared to stick to my word.		
Emotional considerations: I have 3–5 stress-reduction or coping techniques that I use regularly with success.		
A supportive environment: My home is free from distractions so that my child can focus. My child can reach and find all the things they need.		
Believing: I believe my child is capable of learning to be more independent.		
Your support network: I have people that I feel safe leaving my child with. My child works with specialists.		

From *Spectrum of Independence* by Kristin Lombardi and Christine Drew. Copyright © 2025 The Guilford Press. Permission to photocopy this material, or to download enlarged printable versions (*www.guilford.com/lombardi-forms*), is granted to purchasers of this book for personal use; see copyright page for details.

Classifying Stressors

Place all items from the "This is a concern" category into the following categories.

Completely within my control	Somewhat within my control	Completely out of my control

For each of the items in the "completely within my control" and the "somewhat within my control" categories, you can order in priority. Number them according to which you would like to tackle first. Some people might go for the small problems first and then move on to bigger issues, but you may want to work in the opposite direction or tackle more than one at a time. For the things that are completely out of your control, there may be ways to bring the circumstance back into your control, or you may need to wait until the situation has changed or your routine has returned to normal.

From *Spectrum of Independence* by Kristin Lombardi and Christine Drew. Copyright © 2025 The Guilford Press. Permission to photocopy this material, or to download enlarged printable versions (*www.guilford.com/lombardi-forms*), is granted to purchasers of this book for personal use; see copyright page for details.

Brainstorming Solutions

Problem	Solution

Part III

The Basics of Learning

5

"What Do I Need to Know before I Start?"

UNDERSTANDING BEHAVIOR

Diana called out from the living room to the dining room that had been taken over as a playroom for her eight-year-old son Mike, who has autism. "Mike, it's almost time to leave. Let's get going. Can we put on your shoes?" She waited for three breaths before calling out again. "Mike, did you hear me? Come on." She waited again. No response. She sighed and walked into the playroom. Mike was completely engrossed in putting his toy cars into lines on the floor and then crashing the cars together. She got down to his level, said his name again, and then placed her hand over the cars to block his line of sight. He finally looked up. She repeated, "Mike, it's almost time to go. Why don't you put your shoes on?"

Mike began to whine and said, "No no no no, play cars!" Diana took a deep breath and tried a different tactic. "Mike, should we go to the playground? You like the swings. Once you get there, you'll have such a good time." Diana grimaced as Mike continued to verbally protest and lie on top of his cars on the floor. She realized that Mike's favorite shoes were in the car from when he had kicked them off yesterday on the way home from school. She also hadn't packed a bag for the playground (a snack, a sun hat or sunscreen, and water bottle were a must). She decided it wasn't worth it at this point, and said, "Okay, bud, keep playing. We'll try again tomorrow."

If you remember from Chapter 3, problem behavior can be complex, and serious problem behavior requires a behavior analyst to complete assessments and create plans for treatment. What we are addressing in this chapter is how to remedy minor problem behavior such as not listening. Sometimes, a child "not listening" isn't as simple as it sounds. In Diana's situation, we see quite a few issues. First, we have no idea if Mike even heard Diana the first few times she spoke to him. She was in another room and could not tell if she had his attention. Second, he was in the middle of what is probably a highly preferred activity, playing with his cars. For most people, interrupting a preferred activity with no explanation is going to cause some dismay. Third, Diana is asking him to do something that might be difficult, which is putting on his shoes. Who wants to stop doing a fun thing to do a hard thing? Not me.

Fourth, Mike has no idea where he's going once he puts his shoes on, so he has no motivation to complete the routine. Let's assume Mike likes going to the playground. However, even if we like something, it can be hard to stop a preferred activity. Adults struggle with this all the time too. Imagine you're in your bedroom reading a very captivating book, and then suddenly someone is telling you to put on your shoes to go to an unknown location, with no warning. We'd push back on that too! We'd still want to read our book, we'd want more information, and we'd be super annoyed to have to leave the house. In this scenario, there may be many types of motivation at play. The fifth and final issue is that Diana does not follow through on her directions. She makes vague suggestions of what they could do or might do, instead of giving Mike any direct demands. She repeats herself, tries to compromise, and then decides it isn't worth it. This is a very understandable reaction in these situations! But you can probably see how this was all very confusing for Mike and creates a history of being reinforced for not listening to his mother.

But now that you're taking on teaching independent living skills, consistency is key and sticking to your word is critical! That means saying what you mean. Let's look at two behavioral areas you need to be mindful of as a parent—understanding the function of your child's behavior and understanding how the consequences your child receives affect the reoccurrence (or lack thereof) of that behavior.

WTF: What's the Function?

We engage in behavior all day long. Although most people use the term *behavior* to reference things a child is doing that we would prefer they did not do, in the world of behavioral science, behavior is anything we do that can be seen and measured—whether it is "good" or "bad." Have you ever stopped to consider *why* you do a certain behavior? The reason is fairly simple. In general, we engage in behavior because we want to obtain or access something or escape or avoid something. For example, we might get up at 5:30 in the morning because we need to go to work (motivated by obtaining a paycheck), want to meditate (motivated by accessing a mindful state), or want to fit in some extra chores (motivated by avoiding having to do it when everyone is up and vying for your attention). In behavior speak, the "why" behind the behavior is called the function of the behavior. It is the reason we do things.

Much of the time we can determine the function of a behavior with ease. Your child may be clearly motivated by obtaining a reward (eat all veggies to get dessert) or escaping a punishment (staying silent about breaking your favorite mug to avoid getting in trouble). But there are many times when your child might be engaging in minor problem behaviors for which there could be many reasons—or no discernible one! It can be challenging, frustrating, and exhausting. You might ask yourself, "Why does he do that?" By the time you finish this chapter, we want you to reframe that to: "What is the function of his behavior?" When you can understand the function, you can address the problem behavior more skillfully.

Everybody EATS

Once a medical reason has been ruled out (see "Is There a Medical Reason for Your Child's Behavior?" on page 37), you'll want to familiarize yourself with four major categories of functions of behavior. A helpful saying for remembering these functions is "Everybody EATS." EATS stands for *escape, attention, tangible,* and *sensory*. Learning these categories will help you more easily assess what is motivating your child's minor problem behaviors and how to react to them.

And remember earlier you learned that functions are generally either avoiding or obtaining? You'll see these options playing out in some of the categories. For example, you could have a child who is acting out in class to obtain the attention of adults. You could also have a child who is acting out in class because he is trying to get sent to the mindfulness or "cool down" room to escape doing his work. Although both children are acting out, their reasons for doing so are different. It is important to know this because what would reinforce the one child would serve as a punishment for the other. Sending the second child to the mindfulness room would reinforce his behavior—that is exactly what he is hoping the response will be. Sending the first child to the mindfulness room would be the opposite of what he was looking for and might actually serve as deterrent to acting out in class again.

Escape

DEFINITION: When the motivation for engaging in a behavior is to "escape"—that is, to get out of or delay doing something, or to avoid or delay having to be in certain situations, with certain people, or in certain places.

- Joe's mom says, "Time to leave for swimming!" Joe runs to his room and slams the door.
  - Reinforce (encourage): Joe's mom lets him stay in his room.
  - Punish (discourage): Joe's mom goes into his bedroom and helps him get his swimming trunks on.
- Dion's dad says, "Let's get you in the bathtub, bud." Dion lies on the floor and cries.
  - Reinforce (encourage): Dion's dad delays starting the bath routine and says, "Okay, buddy, you don't have to take a bath right now."
  - Punish (discourage): Dion's dad says, "It's time to take a bath. We can watch a movie after," and physically helps Dion to the bathroom to start the bath routine.

Attention

DEFINITION: When the motivation for engaging in a behavior is to attract attention—either good or bad.

- Doris finishes her coloring sheet of her favorite character and shows it to her father.
  - Reinforce (encourage): Doris's father oohs and aahs over it and tells her she did a great job coloring.
  - Punish (discourage): Doris's father does not respond or says, "I'm on the phone, you need to wait."

Understanding Behavior

- Lisa starts crying and screaming because she is frustrated that a toy isn't working.
  - Reinforce (encourage): Lisa's mother runs into the room, makes a fuss about the toy, and fixes it for her.
  - Punish (discourage): Lisa's mother approaches calmly and says, "Come tell me what's wrong." Once Lisa has told her what is wrong, she helps Lisa fix the toy.

Tangible

DEFINITION: When the motivation for a behavior is to obtain a tangible item.

- John cries when his mom tells him that he can't have any more cookies.
  - Reinforce (encourage): John's mom gives him another cookie.
  - Punish (discourage): John's mom tells him that he can have a cookie after dinner if he eats a certain amount of healthy food.
- When Amy's dad turns off the TV, she screams.
  - Reinforce (encourage): Amy's dad turns back on the TV after she screams.
  - Punish (discourage): Amy's dad tells Amy it's time for lunch and helps her walk to the table for lunch.

Sensory

DEFINITION: When the motivation for a behavior is either to avoid or obtain sensory input.

- Jonah hides from his parents in the bathroom when it's time to go to the school play. It's too loud in the auditorium (avoid).
- Jaylin flicks her pen back and forth rapidly in front of her eyes because it feels good to watch it move (obtain).

Sensory stimulation has an internal mechanism of reinforcement, meaning that the feeling of sensory input or relief comes from within the child.

There are accommodations for sensory needs, such as noise-canceling headphones, earplugs, tagless shirts, and many other creative solutions. Parents and the outside world are not the source of reinforcement for behaviors related to the sensory function. Parents can discourage or encourage behaviors that stem from the escape, attention, and tangible functions, but not from the sensory function. Parents can support their child in meeting their sensory needs in an appropriate fashion. This could include teaching coping skills and effective ways to communicate their needs.

These are just some of the countless ways we behave when the function, or reason of a behavior, is to escape, obtain or avoid attention, get something tangible, or meet a sensory need (EATS). And sometimes the function might not be apparent, such as when escaping an internal discomfort like looking for the blanket they've slept with since they were born, or cringing from the feel of socks on their feet. Function is nuanced and every child is different.

The vast majority of behavior is multiply maintained. For example, when you turn off the episode of their favorite TV show and tell your child to brush their teeth (which they hate!) and they begin to cry, they are likely crying due to a combination of trying to escape the demand of brushing their teeth and retaining access to the tangible of their favorite TV show.

Consistency Is Key

Behavioral science shows us that behavior that has been reinforced inconsistently (only some of the time) is actually the hardest to change. Your child has learned that if they hold out long enough, you (or others) might give in. This motivates them to try and "wait you out" to avoid the demand. This is sometimes why therapists or new teachers have an easier time with behavior interventions. The therapists and teachers have no history of giving in to your child.

Of course, most people understand that being a consistent parent is important. We're telling you that being consistent is even more critical for children with disabilities. Learning a skill or a routine may take many more repetitions than it would for a typically developing child. Increasing your consistency increases the likelihood that your child will learn and retain new skills. Your responses drive learning in your child. While typically developing children learn by watching their parents, their peers, and others in their environment, children with autism and other disabilities typically do not pick up as much information from the environment, particularly if it isn't made relevant to them. What they learn needs to be directly taught and requires you to be their primary source of that information.

So, let's turn our attention to several strategies for being consistent in the weeks and months ahead as you work with your child on independence. Again, please return to this chapter as needed; you'll find that certain tips may resonate *after* you've started working through routines.

Say What You Mean

We touched on this topic in Chapter 2, but it's worth repeating. If you mean, "It's 9:00 and time to take a shower. Let's go," *then say that.* Do *not* give the illusion of a suggestion by saying, "Are you ready to take a shower?" Make it a directive, not a question. It helps your child know that your words and actions align. It helps you become a more predictable quantity.

Another issue with these demands dressed up as suggestions is that it opens the door for argument or discussion. Now, of course, asking for extra time or a delay to start a routine can be developmentally appropriate. Your child saying, "Can I have five more minutes?", is great. We all snooze our alarms and we all press "Next Episode" on Netflix sometimes. But some things simply aren't up for negotiation. The ability to negotiate should not be confused with knowing when no means no and it's time to follow directions.

Mean What You Say

We know it's a common phrase, but we really want you to embody "Think before you speak." When parents *don't* think before they speak, and they ask their child to do something they won't or can't do, then the parent's words become meaningless. For example, many parents will offhandedly say to their child with a developmental or intellectual disability, "Say bye to your teacher," knowing full well that their child won't or can't do that. While this demand seems like an innocuous bow to social norms, it's confusing to a child! A child who won't or can't "say bye" verbally learns that what their parent tells them to do is optional, that they don't really mean it. Consider that when the same parent says later, "Okay, get in the car," the child may think that the parent doesn't really mean it! Speaking of social niceties, the teacher also can't stand there for the next two hours while you try to follow through on that demand while your child is on the floor rolling around because they're tired, haven't had a snack, or don't know how to say bye. It's counterproductive for all involved.

Be very careful and think ahead about the consequences of what you say to your child. This means considering all possibilities before you make a demand. Consider your ability to wait it out or help them complete the tasks. If you can't control the environment, or your emotions, enough to keep a demand (perhaps the teacher has to leave so she can't wait for your child to say bye or for you to get frustrated and give up), then don't say it. If you aren't able to enforce what you have told your child to do, then simply don't say it at all. One possible workaround is to give demands that you can help your child complete. If you say, "Wave bye to your teacher," then you can physically help your child wave bye.

You must be able to follow through. This includes being able to stop what you are doing in the moment to help your child follow through with the directive. For example, if you tell your child, "Put the strawberries in the shopping cart," you must be prepared to prompt through the process (we address this in the next chapter) until it's done; in this case you have followed through on meaning what you say. However, if your child physically can't reach into the shopping cart or you are giving your order at the deli counter, then you won't be able to follow through. In these situations, your child learns that you don't really mean what you say. Thinking before you speak gives your words greater value and your child's appraisal of whether you really mean it will change in your favor. You are teaching them that your words are important every time you follow through on what you say.

Finally, you will also need to get others around your child to be on board with meaning what they say as well. We talk about the influence of family in Chapter 4. You may find that some family members will give in to your child at the first sign of resistance. These are not the folks to have around when you try these new ways of interacting with your child. Alternatively, you can ask these family members to read sections (or all) of this book so they can understand the vital importance of follow-through!

Prepare, Prepare, Prepare Some More

As you may have figured out by now, nothing about this process is casual or natural. You will need to think many steps ahead of what you are doing, prepare, think through exactly what you want to say and when to say it, and plan for hiccups and how to handle them. This will be your new normal (or maybe it's always been your normal) that will last until your child becomes independent enough to complete their daily living routines. You know your child best. You know what might cause problem behavior (having to put down a favorite activity to go take a shower), you know where they might get off task (waiting for the water to get to the right temperature), and you know what you can use to make the chore more fun (listening to their favorite music or picking out their favorite pj's to put on afterward). Use that knowledge to plan around these possible issues with each routine and transition. You don't have to start all at once, either. We will ask you to pick one routine to implement these interventions with initially. See if these strategies help your (and your child's) day run more smoothly.

Things May Get Worse before They Get Better . . .

When you begin to stick to your word, mean what you say, and follow through, your child may take some time to adjust. Think about what happens in this scenario: You flip on a light switch and it doesn't work. What do most people do? They flick the light on and off again a few times rapidly. We increase the intensity and frequency of a behavior that works (or used to work, anyway). Then we get creative. We might check the local power station's website to see if there's an outage, or go to our electrical panel to see if we tripped a breaker. We might also call or text a neighbor to see if their lights are out too. In other words, in the short term we intensify our behaviors as we become desperate for the outcome we want (to have light).

In your child's case, their whining may get louder or more frequent, or they may resort to other types of behavior like falling to the floor as they try to get you to give in and let them have their way. This is known as an extinction burst and is a well-researched behavioral phenomenon. So if it happens to you, know that it is quite common and not permanent. There is usually a sharp increase in the intensity or frequency of the problem behavior, followed by a steep decrease—but only if you stay consistent. If you give in, especially when they are having problem behavior, then they learn that they should behave that way in the future (ramping up their problem behavior) to get what they want.

We challenge you to prepare yourself for this eventuality, stick it out, and continue being consistent. Your child may require some additional prompts to get through to the next step. This can feel uncomfortable, but remember that you're asking them to do things that are necessary for their health, well-being, and long-term independence. You are not giving arbitrary instructions, only doing this because of social pressure, or because it's convenient for you.

You can prepare yourself mentally by asking yourself, "What are the best and worst things that can happen from giving my child a directive?" If your child struggles with transitions and you tell your child to go sit at the kitchen table, the worst thing that could happen might be some tears, a red face, maybe a moment on the floor, and then you can help them walk to the table to eat their very favorite lunch. The best that could happen is that you have told your child about the great lunch you have prepared (we'll go over some strategies in just a few paragraphs) and they go to the table eagerly. You won't know until you've tried. And neither will your child. Remember that this way of interacting with you is new for them too. They have expectations that will have to change, and that takes time. And that's totally okay.

If you feel you can't be consistent because of your child's level of problem behavior, please return to Chapter 3 and reassess your child's problem behavior. If you feel you can't be consistent because of your ability to self-regulate, manage outside stressors, or tolerate distress, please return to Chapter 4 and review the suggested ways you can shore yourself up before starting this process.

Manage Your Emotions

Holding a demand can be difficult. Especially if your child is prone to whining or not responding to you. Maintaining a calm voice and tone, neutral facial expression, calm body language, and regular breathing can help manage your own feelings and model self-regulation for your child. If you are huffing and puffing, red-faced, frowning, and tapping your foot in an irritated manner, this can increase your child's reactivity and irritability.

Think about how you want your child to handle difficult situations in the future and be that example. Taking deep breaths, counting to five, and asking for help are all great coping strategies to practice yourself and model for your child. Consistency in your responding helps your child know what is expected of them, how they should behave, and that their whining is not having the effect of upsetting you or getting their way.

Consequences Drive Behavior

Another thing to understand about behavior is that functions are tied to the *consequences* of behavior. In more behavior lingo, a consequence is just something that comes after or as a result of a behavior. All people respond to their environment and the consequences present there. For example, your child saying "Up" results in you picking them up. The consequence of them saying "Up" is that they are lifted up. The consequences you provide to your child are the drivers of your child's behavior. We'll say that again: *The consequences you provide to your child (or that your child receives naturally) are the drivers of your child's behavior.* This is why consistency in your interactions with your child is a must. It is one of the key pillars of effective teaching.

What Is Reinforcement?

As a parent, you're probably pretty sure you know what motivates your child. However, reinforcement is highly personal. What fascinates you may not interest your child. Just because you loved a high five and a "Great job!" doesn't mean your child will. Just because you hated getting a lecture from your parents doesn't mean that your child feels the same way. To truly influence your child's behavior with positive reinforcement, you need to understand what uniquely motivates them.

Take time to observe your child closely and identify their specific interests. Remove your bias from that as much as possible. Notice what engages their attention and brings them joy. Is it encouragement and attention? Access to favorite toys? Being allowed time to do a preferred activity like watching videos of geckos on YouTube? If you want them to finish their homework, is it more effective to promise screen time, a walk to look at the neighbors' new truck, or a visit to a construction zone down the block? Find reinforcement that promotes their unique abilities and values. When in doubt, simply ask them what they find most interesting and see what they're excited about.

Reinforcement versus Punishment

Reinforcement means that the behavior you want to see is closely followed by something that the person finds pleasurable (*positive reinforcement*) or the elimination or removal of something they don't find pleasurable (*negative reinforcement*). Reinforcement increases the likelihood of the behavior happening again in the future. The phrase we use often is *behavior that gets rewarded gets repeated*.

Think about this example. You are in the grocery store. Your child sees something they want but that you don't want to buy. You tell them no. Then before you know it, your child is screaming, lying on the ground, and crying. When you say, "Okay, fine," and hand them the item, they stop crying, and you experience negative reinforcement—you are rewarded by your child not crying and by strangers not staring at you and going back to their shopping (removal of things you find uncomfortable or distressing). Your child is positively reinforced because they got the item they wanted (positive reinforcement). This is a cycle that feeds itself. Many parents find themselves leaving their children at home to avoid just this issue.

Punishment is when a behavior is followed by something the person finds aversive or unpleasant. Positive punishment is not recommended. This could look like going to a loud concert and having a headache as a result, which makes you less likely to go to a concert in the future. Negative punishment would be when siblings fight over a toy and it gets taken away. This may effectively stop the fight over the toy in that moment, however, punishment does not teach a new skill like how to compromise or share toys. The only thing punishment teaches is which specific behaviors not to do. In other words, if your child is creative (as most children are!), then they can find alternative behavior to use. A teacher might say, "Don't call him names," so the next time, the kid sticks his tongue out. While the teacher didn't mean to, she left open the option for the child to try other things to still get the same outcome.

The teacher only told him not to do one of the behaviors. A positive reframing could have sounded like, "Use kind words with yourself and others."

Natural versus Contrived Reinforcement

Some activities have consequences that are less concrete. For things like showering, the reinforcer may not be so clear. As adults, we all shower for different reasons. Some people shower because it feels good to be clean. Others may only shower because they worry that other people can smell them. Still others may shower to keep their hair from getting greasy. These are examples of *natural reinforcement* because they occur as the natural part of the routine. If none of these (or many other reasons) are powerful enough motivation for your child to shower, you may need to add an outside reinforcer, or *contrived reinforcement,* to the routine. *Contrived* just means that someone else—you—are adding the reinforcement rather than reinforcement coming from the routine itself.

Whereas the natural reinforcement for your child putting on their shoes is getting to go to the park (fun!), it gets trickier when the reinforcement isn't built in. Your child may not be naturally reinforced by putting their backpack and shoes away after school in order to keep the house organized, or brushing their teeth so they don't get cavities. Therefore, they may need an additional reinforcer in the early stages of teaching. Contrived reinforcers are just things that you add after they complete a routine. Contrived reinforcers are not directly tied to the routine itself. Getting to watch five minutes of a favorite show after brushing their teeth is an example of contrived reinforcement—the show is not naturally connected to brushing teeth, but it still serves as a reinforcer.

Reinforcement and Punishment in the Real World

To be clear, children with disabilities may not be thinking directly, "Oh, good, Dad gave up, so I'm getting away with this." What is shaping and maintaining their behavior (or keeping the behavior going) are the consequences present in the environment. They might notice, "When I leave my Legos on the floor and ignore Dad's requests to pick them up, Dad gets tired of asking me to pick them up and picks them up himself." Even if they do not make that direct connection, their future behavior responds regardless.

That's the power of consequences. We don't always think about them, but they shape our behavior anyway.

Out in the "real world," consequences are pretty inconsistent. For example, you might get away with speeding on your way home 99 times out of 100, so the one time you get a ticket probably won't really impact your behavior. Yes, paying the fine might sting a little and you might be irritated with yourself, but will it really change your speeding behavior overall? Or will you just be more careful to not speed when you're driving on that one road for the next few weeks? This lack of behavior change is partially because the consequences are inconsistent.

For you and your child, we are striving for long-term behavior change. This requires consistency of reinforcement to learn new skills.

The other reason your behavior might not change is because this is a punishment-based procedure. Punishment-based procedures only focus on decreasing a behavior, not replacing it with something new. So, instead of learning a new skill (like how to plan your morning so you won't be late and need to speed), you just avoid doing the thing that got you in trouble—at least for a little while. Punishment-based procedures might just teach your child to be sneakier about their behavior, just like we tend to only slow down where the speed traps are.

How to Make Reinforcement More Effective

Here are some tips for providing positive reinforcement that is effective, targeted, and clear.

Find reinforcers your child responds to. There is no need to come up with a list of novel or new reinforcers. Instead, view this as your child needing to earn the things that already highly motivate them. Your child should not have access to highly preferred items all day for no reason. Highly preferred items should be viewed as special things that are earned. Why? Because in the real world, no one gets what they want all day for no reason. No one is giving you a paycheck just because you woke up and got out of bed. No one is letting you watch TV all day, every day. We all have things that we need to do in order to access the things we want to do.

Although you do not need to come up with a new list of reinforcers, this could be a good time to try introducing new leisure activities, treats, or privileges to expand your child's repertoire of reinforcers. You can also use this as a place for your child to practice making choices. Giving your child the option to work for time on the iPad or swing is part of increasing their self-determination prerequisite skills. Self-determination, like deciding what activities and foods they enjoy, can help them prepare to make bigger decisions down the road.

Decide what is appropriate for your family and situation. Some families have no problem using small candy or snacks, while other families may not want to use food as a reinforcer. You'll also need to consider the situation and time of day. Providing gummy bears after toothbrushing at night doesn't make sense. Time on the iPad might not be appropriate right before school, because then you need to get it back before putting your child on the bus.

Consider the quantity. Be willing to offer reinforcers at least as often as your child completes the routine. So, for brushing teeth, that's twice a day. For showering, depending on your family, it might be every day or every other day. This also means controlling the "dose" of the reinforcer. You decide how much time on the iPad is appropriate "payment" for completing the task. You can decide how many mini M&M's putting your stuff away after school is worth. And remember, the amount can also be decreased over time slowly as the task gets easier and easier for them. This frees up reinforcers to be used to teach new, more challenging skills.

Control the intensity of the reinforcer. If your child likes attention and praise, you can start by throwing a huge party for their success with whoops, hollers, "Good jobs!", and high fives. You can really lay it on thick. Then you can decrease down to a pat on the back and a smile as the reinforcer over time. You can dial up and down the intensity as needed.

Aim for speedy delivery. The faster your child gets to access the reinforcer following the behavior you want, the better. Research shows that a delay of even a few additional seconds can decrease the speed of learning for some children (Majdalany et al., 2016). This means planning ahead and making sure that the reinforcer is close by, if it's a tangible item, or that you're ready to give your child the attention they have earned after their success. Now, if the reward is to go to the park, then yes, they'll have a slight delay, but we want you to set off to the park immediately. A delay of hours or until "later" won't work in the beginning, and might even hurt your use of reinforcers in the future. Although you can eventually work up to using delayed reinforcement, you want to start with immediate reinforcement. Imagine if your boss told you that you wouldn't get your first paycheck until six months after you started working—how motivated would you be to work? You'd likely be upset, and rightly so.

ACTIVITY: Make a List of Potential Reinforcers

For many children, reinforcement might be getting access to a highly preferred toy, extra playtime with a parent or sibling, or an extra five minutes on the iPad. However, reinforcement might also be a three-minute delay to taking a bath because he's running from you. You running after him and saying "Come back here" might be bonus reinforcement because he's also getting attention or it feels like a game of chase. Whatever you list, make sure you're willing to stock these items or give these privileges at least as often as they are working on the new skill or routine.

We suggest thinking of some reinforcers in each of the following categories for your child:

Tangible—playing video games, climbing on the jungle gym, going for a walk, eating cookies, playing with toys

Sensory—access to kinetic sand, their favorite blanket, music, or sensory activities that involve other people such as big squeezes, being pushed on a swing, tickles

Attention—playing with mommy, being praised by the babysitter for putting their shoes away, making their sibling laugh, getting a high five from dad, eye contact and facial reactions from grandma

Diana and Mike, Take Two

Let's go back to Diana and her son Mike to see how these strategies can be done in real life. Using the strategies we went over in "How to Make Reinforcement More Effective," here's how we would suggest Diana handle the situations she was facing.

Diana started giving Mike a rundown of the day at breakfast. She knew it was important to tell Mike in advance of what was going to happen. She knew that increasing the predictability of his schedule would help him handle the transition from playing to putting on his shoes. "Mike, this morning we are going to the playground. What do you like to do at the playground?" Mike replied, "Swings! And sandbox!" Diana responded, "That's right! I can push you on the swings if you want. I think it will be really fun." Next, she stated the exact plan for the morning that she would stick to: "We're going to eat breakfast, then you can play for 30 minutes, and then we need to put on your shoes to go to the playground. Sound good?" Mike nodded vigorously.

Diana used the next 15 minutes that Mike played by himself to get some things done in the kitchen. About 15 minutes before it was time to leave, Diana went into the playroom. She got down on Mike's level, made sure he was attending to her by asking a few simple questions, and then told him, "Okay, buddy, we've got 15 more minutes. I'm setting a timer." Using timers was new for her, but they'd been amazing for helping Mike understand the passage of time. They'd purchased a visual timer that showed the time counting down. Diana returned to gain his attention and then remind Mike at 5 minutes from the time to leave, "You can play for 5 more minutes." While he played, she prepared. She gathered all the items needed to go to the playground and put them in a bag. This way the difficult part (putting on Mike's shoes) would be the only delay to leaving. She returned to the playroom with 1 minute left on the timer, with Mike's favorite (and least difficult to get on) shoes in her hand. When the timer went off, she got his attention again and said, "Great job playing by yourself, Mike. We're going to the playground so you can play on the swings. Do you want to take three cars or five cars to the playground with you?" Mike responded, "Five cars!" Diana said, "Great idea, pick five." Mike carefully selected five cars and Diana had him put them in the bag she had packed for the playground. Diana said, "Time for shoes. First shoes, then playground." Mike put his shoes on, and they headed for the car.

You may read this scenario and think phew, that's a ton of work just to go to the playground. And yes, at first it will be extra work. However, once your child gets used to the framework of following your lead, and you get the extra practice at following through, these strategies can be faded, or your child can take charge of them. There's no reason Mike can't start setting his own timers and use a script of reminders to keep himself on track like, "I'm putting on my shoes so we can go to the playground. I'm going to swing on the swings."

ACTIVITY: Am I Ready to Support Behavior Change?

Please answer the self-efficacy questions below to self-assess how confident you are in your ability to support your child's behavior change using the strategies noted earlier. Please rate yourself from 1 to 5 using the following guidelines:

1 = I never do this.
2 = I do this every once in a while.
3 = I probably do this about half the time.
4 = I do this the majority of the time.
5 = I do this 100% of the time.

Before you begin implementing any of our suggestions, rate yourself here. Then, give yourself one week of implementing these strategies to the best of your ability in one or two routines and return to see if your score has changed.

Parent statements	Rating time 1	Rating time 2
I set up the environment before giving my child a demand.		
I plan ahead to make sure my child is prepared for when I give demands.		
I stick to my word. If I say something to my child, I follow through.		
I keep myself calm when my child is upset.		
I model calm behavior for my child to help them self-regulate.		
Total		

Thinking about how your behavior impacts your child's behavior can be a delicate dance. Following through is important, but even more important is to only tell your child to do things that you can follow through on. Think of your words like a pact or a promise. When you are speaking to your child, you are promising that you mean what you say and that you've said what you mean. You're also promising that you've done everything you can to set your child up for success before the demand comes. Kept promises build trust, while broken ones may leave your child feeling uncertain. You are the most powerful source of change in your child's life. Build up that trust so that when you ask them to do a hard thing, they know that they can.

6

"How Am I Going to Teach?"
EMPOWERING VERSUS ENABLING

Doug was in a rush to get his 11-year-old son Tommy out to the school bus and himself off to work. He had a big meeting that day, so he did not want Tommy to miss the bus. If they didn't get out there on time, the bus would only wait a minute or two before it took off, and Tommy's school was a 20-minute drive in the opposite direction of Doug's office. Doug called for Tommy to come to the entryway and sit on the bottom step of the stairs. Tommy came over, sat down on the step, and waited for Doug to put his shoes on for him. Doug knew that Tommy should be putting on his own shoes at this point. Worse yet, he was pretty sure that Tommy was capable of putting his shoes on himself, but Tommy was so used to having it done for him that he never even attempted to do it himself. Doug knew the only way that Tommy would start putting on his own shoes was if he showed Tommy how to do it and stopped doing it for him. Doug made a mental note that he needed to carve out time to teach Tommy to put on his own shoes and allot more time in the morning so Tommy would have time to practice, but today was definitely not the day to start.

If you're around young kids often, there's a fun developmental phase that includes a lot of "I do that!", "Sammy do it!", or "Me do it by myself!" where young children insist on doing things on their own. Typically developing children also begin to experience embarrassment and develop a desire for privacy when adults are, for instance, helping them in the bathroom. Often neurodiverse children experience this phase later in life, if at all. This means parents are missing out on the cue from their child that it's time for them to back off and let their child complete the task themselves.

In addition to a delayed desire for privacy and independence, neurodiverse children often have other delays in the areas of motor skills, cognition, and attention. These delays make completing daily tasks more challenging, so naturally, we step in to help. Sometimes, though, with the best of intentions, we tend to *over*help, either by embedding ourselves into their daily routines or by doing the activities of the routine for them. This makes both their life and our life easier—in the short run—by ensuring we get out of the house on time, prevent a tantrum, or make sure they wash behind their ears. Over time, though, it becomes a habit for us to do things for them, instead of teaching them to do things for themselves. This habit gets parents and their child stuck in an enabling and overhelping cycle, which over time leads to older children still needing the assistance and attention typically reserved for a much younger child.

Refraining from Overhelping

A critical concept you will learn during the course of this book is to become aware of situations where you are enabling your child rather than encouraging them to be more independent. In these cases, you make your child more dependent on you, rather than less dependent. Subtle shifts in how you assist your child during a daily living activity can be the difference between creating further dependence on you or teaching your child to depend on themselves. This book will show you how to recognize when you are overhelping. We will teach you alternate interactions to use with your child that will not only increase their independence over time, but also decrease your need to be involved in the activity. Long term, this gives your child the opportunity to care for their own basic needs, and you the peace of mind to know that they will not be dependent on others to do those things for them for the rest of their life.

You probably just call it helping, but in clinical practice we refer to assistance or cues used to encourage the use of a specific skill a *prompt*. Prompts work as a teaching tool because they allow you to provide the minimum amount of support needed in order for your child to complete the activity. This allows them to build muscle memory and incrementally add on new skills to the skills they already can do independently. The next step to increase your child's independence is learning how to recognize the types of prompts you use with your child and the frequency with which you use them.

Just like reinforcement, the quicker you deliver a prompt, the better. This allows the routine to follow a natural timing and flow, and decreases wait time during the acquisition or learning phase. Wait time during learning may lead to frustration, or your child engaging in off task or repetitive behavior between steps in the routine. Ultimately, the most transformative step of prompts is learning how to *fade* them, or incrementally decrease them until they are no longer needed. We refer to this as *prompt fading*. This is the step that allows you to systematically fade the prompts so that your child can learn how to successfully complete each task on their own. You will learn how to fade prompts in Chapter 8.

The purpose of a prompt is to assist someone in doing something better. The purpose of prompt fading is to teach someone to do something more independently. So, we are using prompts and prompt fading to teach your child how to do things for themselves, instead of you doing it for them. The key being *"Let me teach you"* rather than *"Let me do it for you."* There is a big difference here. Teaching a skill to your child means you are giving them the tool to do that skill independently. Doing something for your child every day means they will always be reliant on you to do it for them. This can lead to *prompt dependency*—a situation where your child has become dependent on your presence, feedback, and assistance to complete an activity. The ability to skillfully fade your prompts, and eventually your presence, out of the routine is a very important step to increasing your child's independence. You'll learn more about prompt dependency and fading of prompts in Chapter 8. So, let's dive in to the different types of prompts!

Types of Prompts

Physical Prompts

DEFINITION: A type of prompt where the parent is physically assisting the child to complete a task; these are the most intrusive types of prompts, require close proximity, and necessitate physical contact to deliver.

EXPLANATION: This is not the same thing as doing the task for your child. When using a physical prompt, you are placing your hands on their body and guiding them to complete the task.

MOST-TO-LEAST PROMPT HIERARCHY:

Hand-over-hand (HOH) prompt, also known as a full physical (FP) prompt

Partial physical (PP) prompt: This can occur at different body parts, for example, a partial physical prompt at the wrist (PP at wrist), then the elbow, then the shoulder

Independent (I): The child completes the task without support

EXAMPLES:

HOH/FP: You place your hands over your child's hands and prompt him to put his pants on by guiding his hands and fingers to grasp the pants by the waistband.

PP at wrist: You place your hands over your child's wrists and prompt him to put his pants on, guiding his hands where they need to go, but not prompting his fingers, and your child does the grasping portion of the task on his own.

PP at elbows: You place your hands over your child's elbows and prompt him to put his pants on, guiding his arms where they need to go, but not prompting his hands or fingers.

PP at shoulder: You place your hands on your child's shoulders to turn him in the direction of his pants so that he picks them up and puts them on independently.

I: He walks over to his pants and puts them on himself.

Abbreviations for Physical Prompts

Abbreviation	Meaning
HOH/FP	Hand-over-hand/Full physical prompt
PP	Partial physical prompt
I	Independent

WHEN TO USE: You use physical prompts when teaching your child how to complete a motor task that they do not know how to complete on their own; examples include toothbrushing, dressing, cutting food, washing their hands, and wiping themselves after using the toilet.

How Intrusive Are Your Prompts?

It's important to note that prompts exist on a spectrum. On one side, we have the *most intrusive* prompts, which are *physical prompts*. That is where you are actually making physical contact with your child. On the other end of the spectrum, we have our *least intrusive* prompts, which are *visual prompts,* or things that your child can see in their environment.

In the real world, intrusive prompts are much less appropriate as children age. Think about holding a 20-year-old's hands under the faucet in a public bathroom. The goal is to use the least intrusive prompt possible while still having your child be successful at the task. Less intrusive prompts are also easier to fade. We know it seems like we're jumping ahead, but we always plan with the end in mind. The end goal is for your child to do these tasks as independently as possible, so fading prompts is at the forefront of that planning.

Model Prompts

DEFINITION: A type of prompt where you do the action so your child can watch you and use you as a model for what they are supposed to do; these are less intrusive prompts, can be delivered at an increased distance, and do not require physical contact to deliver.

MOST-TO-LEAST PROMPT HIERARCHY:

Full model prompt (FMP): You model the entire action.

Partial model prompt (PMP): You model part of the action.

Independent (I): The child completes the action following a verbal cue or an environmental prompt, or because they know it is the next part of a sequence.

EXAMPLES:

FMP: You want your child to put their toys away and have given the verbal directive once already. Your child has not responded. You gain their attention, then give the verbal directive a second time and pair it with you modeling putting the toys away. Your child begins to put the toys away.

PMP: You want your child to put their toys away and have given a verbal directive once already. Your child has not responded to the initial directive. You give the verbal directive a second time and this time pair it with you bending over to pick up a toy. When your child sees you reach for the toy, he begins to pick up and put away the toys.

I: You want your child to put their toys away; you give the verbal directive once and they put their toys away—no model prompt is needed.

WHEN TO USE: Use model prompts when your child is physically capable of completing a task, but they have not seen the step before; for example, if you buy a new shampoo dispenser for the shower, you would model (show them) how to press the button. You would only use a model prompt if a less intrusive gestural prompt was not enough.

Abbreviations for Model Prompts

Abbreviation	Meaning
FMP	Full model prompt
PMP	Partial model prompt
I	Independent

Gestural Prompts

DEFINITION: A prompt where you point to an item or location that is needed to complete an activity; these are less intrusive than the previous types of prompts, are easier to deliver, and do not always require close proximity.

MOST-TO-LEAST PROMPT HIERARCHY: The way to fade a gestural prompt is to increase your distance from the item you are pointing to. The abbreviation for a gestural prompt is GP.

EXAMPLES:

More intrusive prompt: Your child is supposed to be brushing his teeth and has entered the bathroom, but starts to engage in off-task behavior; you touch his toothbrush with your pointer finger and he begins the toothbrushing sequence.

Less intrusive prompt: Your child is supposed to be brushing his teeth and has entered the bathroom, but starts to engage in off-task behavior; you point to his toothbrush from the doorway of the bathroom, and he begins the toothbrushing sequence.

WHEN TO USE: Your child knows how to physically complete the activity but has become sidetracked; they do not need a model prompt, but just a reminder of what they are supposed to be doing or where they are supposed to be.

Positional Prompts

DEFINITION: A prompt where you put the needed item to complete an activity in a more convenient location than it would naturally be; this is a less intrusive prompt type, can be set up before the routine takes place, and is similar to the prompts available in the natural environment.

MOST-TO-LEAST PROMPT HIERARCHY: Similar to gestural prompts, the way to fade positional prompts is by changing the distance, only this time, you are decreasing the distance from where the item should be naturally located until your child is able to complete the task without you needing to move the item at all. There is no set abbreviation for a positional prompt, but we like to use P @ [location] so we know where the therapist or parent is in relation to the child. For example, P @ edge of vanity or P @ foot of bed.

EXAMPLES: Leaving your child's toothbrush on the vanity next to the sink, instead of in the toothbrush holder; laying your child's clothes out on the bed; leaving your child's vitamin on the table next to their breakfast.

WHEN TO USE: Positional prompts are great to use when your child needs a visual reminder of what they are supposed to do or when you are not ready to teach them the skills they need in order to complete that step independently. For example, if you are working on having your child get themselves dressed independently in the morning, you likely will not want to also include having them pick out their outfit at the same time. You could use the positional prompt of leaving the clothes out for them until they know how to dress themselves independently, and then teach them how to pick out their own outfit as the next step.

Visual Prompts

DEFINITION: Any prompt that provides a visual cue for what the child is supposed to be doing. Activity schedules, also known as visual schedules, fall into this category. These can be added to the environment artificially, or you can rely on the visuals present in the natural environment. Although visual schedules can be a great tool, we do not discuss them in detail, as an explanation of the proper creation and fading of a visual schedule requires more depth then can be addressed in this book.

MOST-TO-LEAST PROMPT HIERARCHY: There are different ways to fade a visual prompt. The picture can be faded brightness wise, its size can be decreased, or it can be replaced with a word. There is no set abbreviation for visual prompts, but we use Vis P.

WHEN TO USE: In relation to daily living routines, visual prompts can be used for a child who has trouble remembering where something is or how to complete all steps in a sequence.

EXAMPLES: Creating a picture schedule of your child's morning routine, taping a picture of a shirt on their shirt drawer, writing a to-do list for your day.

Verbal Prompts

Verbal prompts are a type of prompt where the parent is verbally directing or assisting the child to complete a task. Verbal prompts are the most common type of prompt—you probably use them dozens of times a day (or even within a few minutes if trying to get out the door!). Yet, they're also the type of prompt most often misused by well-meaning parents. We'll help you understand the different forms of verbal prompts, when to use them, and how.

Verbal prompts take two forms: (1) those used when running a verbal program, and (2) those used when running a daily routine or task analysis.

A verbal program uses verbal prompts to teach language and communication skills to a child. Verbal prompting in a verbal program might be used to teach your child to fill in the last word of a song, answer "Wh" questions, or respond to a comment to continue a conversation—all in an effort to teach your child to develop their own communication skills. This is the appropriate use of a verbal prompt.

In contrast, verbal prompting in a daily routine or task analysis is used to keep your child on task. These verbal prompts take the form of reminders or encouragement. Although this may sound quite helpful—"Stevie, remember to hang up your jacket" or "You're almost done, just one more toy to put away!"—this is an inappropriate use of a verbal prompt. Yes, that's right, verbal prompts when teaching your child how to be independent can be more hindering than helpful, because they have the potential to make your child more, not less, dependent on you.

Let's break this down. As mentioned, within the context of a daily living routine, we view verbal prompts as reminders. Although we all need reminders at times, you do not want your voice embedded into your child's routines, as your voice is the hardest thing to fade. That being said, your child is not a mind reader, so there will be times when you need to give them verbal directions. The key is to know when to give those directions and when to use a different type of prompt instead.

Here are a few examples of when you would want to give your child verbal directions: (1) You want your child to pick up their toys and there is no other cue to notify them of this, such as a TV show ending; (2) you want your child to do something for the first time, like put their plate in the sink when they finish their breakfast; (3) you want your child to get ready to go out and they do not have the skills to tell time yet. These are all situations where your child needs information in order to know what to do next—so giving a verbal direction is warranted.

This is different from using a verbal prompt in a situation where your child should know what comes next. In such instances, a nonverbal prompt is preferred. Let's look at slightly modified examples from earlier, where we want to avoid using a verbal prompt: (1) You are teaching your child to clean up their toys when their TV show ends as part of their evening routine; in this case, the end of the TV show is the directive to start cleaning up the toys. (2) You have already taught your child how to put their breakfast plates in the sink and are now teaching them to do it independently once they finish their breakfast. (3) Your child will go upstairs to shower if you tell them, but now you are teaching them to do so when an alarm on their phone goes off. The difference is that, in these cases, you are transferring the prompt from your voice to another cue in the environment.

Worried that you've been doing it all wrong? That's okay! The purpose of this book is to teach you how to teach your child to be independent. You'll replace verbal prompts with more effective prompts, which you will learn in the remainder of this chapter. You're doing great—and you'll be doing even better after you learn how to replace your verbal prompts with prompts that can be more easily faded.

ACTIVITY: Identify the Prompts

VIGNETTE 1

Directions

Following is the vignette about Jamie and Taylor from Chapter 1. It is an example of a child being prompted through the wake-up and dressing part of his morning routine. It illustrates a parent who is unknowingly prompting their child inappropriately and a child who has become prompt dependent. Incorrectly using prompts is inefficient because they do not set the stage for teaching new skills and eventual fading of the prompts to teach independence. This is a common scenario of a parent doing the best they can despite having not received any instruction on prompting. As you read through the vignette, underline each of the prompts that Taylor gives Jamie. Then, using the chart on the facing page, classify each prompt into its proper category.

"Jamie, time to wake up," Taylor whispers to her son. This is the third round of wake-ups she's tried with Jamie this morning. He grumbles and rolls over. She picks him up and places him on his feet. He rubs his eyes and sits on the floor. Taylor says, "Time to potty." Jamie is eight years old and has an intellectual disability. Jamie stays on the floor until Taylor lifts him to standing again. She points toward the bathroom and says, "Go potty." Jamie walks to the bathroom, still rubbing his eyes and yawning. He uses the bathroom and comes back into his bedroom. Taylor says, "I didn't hear the flush. Go flush the toilet and wash your hands." Jamie goes back and flushes the toilet, but returns before washing his hands. She says, "Hands," and points to the bathroom again, sending him back in to wash his hands. He comes back with wet hands that don't smell like soap, and water down the front of his sleep shirt. Not having the energy to send him back a third time, Taylor moves on to the next part of the routine. She points to Jamie's outfit that she laid out on the bed while he was in the bathroom. "Time to get dressed. It's picture day today." Jamie stands next to the clothes and looks at Taylor. Taylor says, "Okay, take your sleep shirt and pants off." Jamie is back on the floor again, tugging at his slightly-too-small pj pants. Taylor gets out her phone and adds "new pj's for Jamie" to her Target shopping list. Since he's having a hard time, she helps him pull his pj pants off and makes up a silly song about being stuck like a snug little bug in a rug.

Jamie laughs. The sleep shirt is also a challenge to get over his head, so Jamie walks over to her and says "Help" as he is trying to get the shirt over his head. Taylor steps in to help again by pulling his shirt over his head. Taylor then proceeds to tell Jamie to get dressed two times, points to two specific articles of clothing to keep him on task, points to his underwear to make sure he puts them on before he puts on his pants, and holds him steady while he puts one leg and then the other into underwear and then again for his pants. Using her sing-song voice, she tells him about the delicious breakfast she'll make for him, and tells him "Arms up!" before putting on his new shirt. Taylor puts Jamie's wet pj's into the hamper in Jamie's room and says, "Let's go eat breakfast!"

Classify each of the prompts you found into this chart to see the frequency with which each prompt was used.

Type of prompt	Frequency
Full physical prompts	
Partial physical prompts	
Verbal prompts	
Gestural prompts	
Model prompts	
Positional prompts	
Tasks that Taylor did for Jamie instead of prompting him to do them	
Total prompts	

Answer Key for Vignette 1

"Jamie, time to wake up," Taylor whispers to her son (*verbal prompt*). This is the third round of wake-ups she's tried with Jamie this morning. (*So technically this would be 3 verbal prompts.*) He grumbles and rolls over. She picks him up and places him on his feet (*full physical prompt*). He rubs his eyes and sits on the floor. Taylor says, "Time to potty" (*verbal prompt*). Jamie is eight years old and has an intellectual disability. Jamie stays on the floor until

Taylor lifts him to standing again (*full physical prompt*). She points toward the bathroom (*gestural prompt*) and says, "Go potty" (*verbal prompt*). Jamie walks to the bathroom, still rubbing his eyes and yawning. He uses the bathroom and comes back into his bedroom. Taylor says, "I didn't hear the flush. Go flush the toilet and wash your hands" (*verbal prompt*). Jamie goes back and flushes the toilet, but returns before washing his hands. She says, "Hands" (*partial verbal prompt*), and points to the bathroom again (*gestural prompt*), sending him back in to wash his hands. He comes back with wet hands that don't smell like soap, and water down the front of his sleep shirt. (*There is no additional prompt here, but note that he did not complete the task of handwashing at an acceptable level of proficiency.*) Not having the energy to send him back a third time, Taylor moves on to the next part of the routine. She points to Jamie's outfit (*gestural prompt*) that she laid out on the bed while he was in the bathroom (*positional prompt*). "Time to get dressed. (*verbal prompt*) It's picture day today." Jamie stands next to the clothes and looks at Taylor (*positional prompt*). Taylor says, "Okay, take your sleep shirt and pants off" (*verbal prompt*). Jamie is back on the floor again, tugging at his slightly-too-small pj pants. Taylor gets out her phone and adds "new pj's for Jamie" to her Target shopping list. (*This is an example of the environment making the routine more difficult for Jamie to function independently; when and how to accommodate your child are discussed in Chapter 9.*) Since he's having a hard time, she helps him pull his pj pants off (*partial physical prompt*) and makes up a silly song about being stuck like a snug little bug in a rug (*although not a prompt, this would be considered social reinforcement in the form of attention*) Jamie laughs. The sleep shirt is also a challenge to get over his head, so Jamie walks over to her and says "Help" as he is trying to get the shirt over his head. Taylor steps in to help again by pulling his shirt over his head (*partial physical prompt*). Taylor then proceeds to tell Jamie to get dressed two times (*2 verbal prompts*), points to two specific articles of clothing to keep him on task (*2 gestural prompts*), points to his underwear to make sure he puts them on before he puts on his pants (*gestural prompt*), holding him steady while he puts one leg and then the other into underwear and then again for his pants (*2 partial physical prompts*), using her sing-song voice, telling him about the delicious breakfast she'll make for him (*although not a prompt, this would be considered an ineffective use of reinforcement due to the delivery*), and tells him "Arms up!" (*verbal prompt*) before putting on his new shirt (*not a prompt, as she did it for him*). Taylor puts Jamie's wet pj's into the hamper in Jamie's room (*again, not a prompt as she did it for him*) and says, "Let's go eat breakfast!" (*verbal prompt*).

Now compare how many of each type of prompt Taylor used during the routine to how many you found, using the chart below.

Prompts that Taylor used	How many I found
Full physical prompts–2	
Partial physical prompts–4	
Verbal prompts–14	
Gestural prompts–6	
Model prompts–0	
Positional prompts–2	
Tasks that Taylor did for Jamie–2	
Total prompts–30	

Wow! Taylor probably feels exhausted, and she hasn't even finished getting Jamie ready for school yet. Now they will head downstairs to have breakfast, pack his snack and lunch, brush his teeth, put on his jacket, and get his backpack before heading out to the bus. It is reasonable to assume that Taylor is likely prompting Jamie well over 100 times before he has even left for school in the morning. The positive piece of this is that there is a lot of room for improvement—even if Taylor can decrease the prompts she is using by half, it would increase Jamie's independence level and make her morning easier.

VIGNETTE 2

Directions

This vignette looks at Jamie's morning routine shortly after Taylor has learned about the different types of prompts, which types of prompts are most effective when teaching a daily living routine, and the importance of fading the prompts so that Jamie can learn to complete the routine independently. This time you will see an example of a parent who is consciously prompting her child when needed, noting the prompts she is using, and being mindful of steps where she can begin to fade her prompts. As you read through the vignette, underline each of the prompts that Taylor gives Jamie. Then, using the chart on the facing page, classify each prompt into its proper category.

"Jamie, time to wake up," Taylor whispers to her son. Taylor learned from her parent trainer that verbal prompts are the hardest to fade, so instead of repeatedly asking Jamie to get up, she waits a few seconds to see if he responds, and when he doesn't, she physically prompts him out of bed by picking him up and placing him on his feet. He rubs his eyes and sits on the floor. Taylor lifts him to stand again, orients him toward the bathroom by placing her hands on his shoulders and turning him, and points to the bathroom. Jamie walks to the bathroom, still rubbing his eyes and yawning. Taylor follows him to the bathroom so that if he needs any prompts while he is in there, she can immediately prompt him before he moves on to the next step. Jamie uses the bathroom and steps away before flushing. Taylor points to the flusher on the toilet. Jamie turns around and flushes the toilet, but then starts to walk toward the door before washing his hands. Taylor points to the sink, cueing him to wash his hands. Taylor bought a kid-friendly soap pump that is easier for Jamie to use and cleared all the unnecessary items off the vanity so that the only things out are the soap, Jamie's toothbrush, and toothpaste. She also keeps the soap closer to the edge instead of all the way back, as Jamie has to really reach to get the soap when it is in the usual position. It turns out that once these changes were made, Jamie was able to independently wash his hands. Taylor points to Jamie's outfit that she laid out on the bed before she woke him up. Jamie does not walk toward his clothes but instead heads to the window. Taylor says, "Time to get dressed," but then remembers she should have used a physical prompt to orient him toward his clothes instead of a verbal prompt. Taylor refrains from mentioning that it is the 100th day of school celebration today, as she knows the eventual goal is to fade her presence from the routine. She instead holds off, knowing that there will be time to talk during breakfast. Jamie stands next to the clothes and looks at Taylor. Taylor looks away so as not to provide any unnecessary cues. She waits a few seconds to see if Jamie starts to get undressed on his own. When he does not, Taylor takes his hand and hooks his thumb into the waist of his pants. Taylor has replaced Jamie's tight pajamas with looser pajamas that are easier for him to get on and off. He can now take his pants and shirt off by himself. Taylor then physically orients Jamie to his clothes to get him to initiate getting dressed. She points to his underwear to make sure he puts them on before he puts on his pants, and physically prompts him to sit on the floor instead of holding him steady while he puts in one leg and then the other. Jamie independently stands to pull up his underwear and then independently sits again to put on his pants. Taylor has stopped telling him about the delicious breakfast she'll make for him as a way to keep him on task and instead plans to give him his favorite fidget toy once he's ready to go downstairs. She takes his hands and prompts him through the process of putting on his shirt. Taylor waits to see if Jamie remembers to put his pj's into the hamper, but when he heads toward the door instead, she orients him toward the pajamas and points to them. He puts the pj's in the hamper. Taylor meets Jamie at the bedroom door and praises him for doing a great job with this part of his morning routine. She lets him know that he earned his fidget toy, and then they head downstairs for breakfast.

Classify each of the prompts you found into this chart to see the frequency with which each prompt was used.

Type of prompt	Frequency
Full physical prompts	
Partial physical prompts	
Verbal prompts	
Gestural prompts	
Model prompts	
Positional prompts	
Tasks that Taylor did for Jamie instead of prompting him to do them	
Total prompts	

Answer Key for Vignette 2

"Jamie, time to wake up," Taylor whispers to her son (*verbal prompt*). Taylor learned from her parent trainer that verbal prompts are the hardest to fade, so instead of repeatedly asking Jamie to get up, she waits a few seconds to see if he responds, and when he doesn't, she physically prompts him out of bed by picking him up and placing him on his feet (*full physical prompt*).

He rubs his eyes and sits on the floor. Taylor lifts him to stand again (*full physical prompt*), orients him toward the bathroom by placing her hands on his shoulders and turning him (*partial physical prompt*), and points to the bathroom (*gestural prompt*). Jamie walks to the bathroom, still rubbing his eyes and yawning. Taylor follows him to the bathroom so that if he needs any prompts while he is in there, she can immediately prompt him before he moves on to the next step. Jamie uses the bathroom and steps away before flushing. Taylor points to the flusher on the toilet (*gestural prompt*). Jamie turns around and flushes the toilet, but then starts to walk toward the door before washing his hands. Taylor points to the sink (*gestural prompt*), cueing him to wash his hands. Taylor bought a kid-friendly soap pump that is easier for Jamie to use (*accommodation*), and cleared all the unnecessary items off the vanity so that the only things out are the soap, Jamie's toothbrush, and toothpaste (*not a prompt but an environmental accommodation*). She also keeps the soap closer to the edge instead of all the way back (*positional prompt*), as Jamie has to really reach to get the soap when it is in the usual position. It turns out that once these changes were made, Jamie was able to independently wash his hands. Taylor points to Jamie's outfit (*gestural prompt*) that she laid out on the bed before she woke him up (*positional prompt*). Jamie does not walk toward his clothes but instead heads to the window. Taylor says, "Time to get dressed" (*verbal prompt*), but then remembers she should have used a physical prompt to orient him toward his clothes instead of a verbal prompt. Taylor refrains from mentioning it is the 100th day of school celebration today, as she knows the eventual goal is to fade her presence from the routine. She instead holds off, knowing that there will be time to talk during breakfast. Jamie stands next to the clothes and looks at Taylor. Taylor looks away so as not to provide any unnecessary cues. She waits a few seconds to see if Jamie starts to get undressed on his own. When he does not, Taylor takes his hand and hooks his thumb into the waist of his pants (*partial physical prompt*). Taylor has replaced Jamie's pajamas with looser pajamas that are easier for him to get on and off (*accommodation—discussed in Chapter 9*). He can now take his pants and shirt off by himself. Taylor then physically orients Jamie to his clothes to get him to initiate getting dressed (*partial physical prompt*). She points to his underwear to make sure he puts them on before he puts on his pants (*gestural prompt*), and physically prompts him to sit on the floor to put on his underwear (*partial physical prompt*) instead of holding him steady while he puts in one leg and then the other. Jamie independently stands to pull up his underwear and then independently sits again to put on his pants. Taylor has stopped telling him about the delicious breakfast she'll make for him as a way to keep him on task, and instead plans to give him his favorite fidget toy once he's ready to go downstairs (*appropriate use of reinforcement following completion of the routine instead of relying on bribing him during the routine; immediate reinforcement*). She takes his hands and prompts him through the process of putting on his shirt (*full physical/hand-over-hand prompt*). Taylor waits to see if Jamie remembers to put his pj's into the hamper, but when he heads to the door instead, she orients him toward the pajamas (*partial physical prompt*) and points to them (*gestural prompt*). He puts the pj's in the hamper. Taylor meets Jamie at the bedroom door and praises him for doing a great job with this part of his morning routine. She lets him know that he earned his fidget toy, and then they head downstairs for breakfast.

Now compare how many of each type of prompt Taylor used during the routine (see the table below) to how many you found.

Prompts that Taylor used	How many I found
Full physical prompts—3	
Partial physical prompts—5	
Verbal prompts—2	
Gestural prompts—6	
Model prompts—0	
Positional prompts—2	
Tasks that Taylor did for Jamie—0	
Total prompts—18	

Although Taylor is still involved in the routine and maintaining close physical proximity to Jamie, she is in a much better position to fade herself from the routine. She has drastically decreased her use of verbal prompts and replaced them with physical and gestural prompts, both of which are easier to fade than verbal prompts. Additionally, by accommodating Jamie with larger pajamas, a new soap dispenser, and reorganizing the environment, Jamie needed significantly fewer prompts overall to complete the routine.

VIGNETTE 3

Directions

This vignette looks back in on Jamie and Taylor a few weeks into Taylor's parent training sessions. Taylor started video recording the morning routine so she could watch it and get clear on how and when she was prompting Jamie. Her parent trainer taught her how to create a task analysis for the morning routine (which you will learn in the next chapter) and score each step of the routine. In this vignette, Taylor has started to fade her prompts as well as her presence during parts of the routine. As you read through the vignette, underline each of the prompts that Taylor gives Jamie. Then, using the chart on the facing page, classify each prompt into its proper category.

> Jamie's child-friendly alarm clock starts to play his favorite song when it is time for him to get out of bed. The alarm clock has replaced the need for Taylor to verbally prompt Jamie to get out of bed in the morning. Taylor watches by the doorway to see if Jamie gets up by himself. The song ends and Jamie is still in bed, so she walks to the bed and prompts him to sit up by tapping his shoulder. Jamie gets out of bed and heads to the bathroom. Taylor goes back to the bedroom doorway but continues to listen to ensure that Jamie is following all the steps of the bathroom routine. Jamie uses the bathroom, steps away before flushing, and turns on the faucet to wash his hands. Taylor steps into the bathroom and points to the flusher on the toilet. Jamie goes back to flush the toilet, and then heads back to the sink to wash his hands. Since the accommodations were put in place with the easier soap pump and the cleared-off vanity, Jamie can now complete the handwashing part of the routine independently. Jamie walks out of the bathroom and toward his clothes. Taylor remains in the bedroom doorway because she knows Jamie is now able to take his pajamas off independently. After taking his pajamas off, Jamie sits on the floor to put on his underwear—only he is about to put them on backwards. Taylor steps in and points to the front of the underwear. Jamie then proceeds to put on his underwear and then his pants. Taylor has asked the physical therapist at school to work with Jamie on putting his pants on without needing to sit on the floor. After putting on his pants, Jamie starts to wander away from the rest of his clothes, so Taylor steps in again and points to his clothes. Although Jamie sometimes still requires prompts to stay on task, the overall number of prompts he needs to complete this part of the morning routine is significantly less than what it had been only a few weeks ago. Taylor knows Jamie still needs some

assistance with putting on his shirt, so she stays close by and steps in when needed to guide Jamie's hands to the sleeve holes. Once his shirt is on, Taylor knows he can independently put on his socks and put his clothes in the hamper, so she heads down the hall toward the top of the stairs. Jamie finishes up his routine and meets Taylor at the top of the stairs. Taylor praises him for doing a great job with this part of his morning routine, gives him his favorite fidget toy, and then they head down to breakfast.

Classify each of the prompts you found into this chart to see the frequency with which each prompt was used.

Type of prompt	Frequency
Full physical prompts	
Partial physical prompts	
Verbal prompts	
Gestural prompts	
Model prompts	
Positional prompts	
Tasks that Taylor did for Jamie instead of prompting him to do them	
Total prompts	

Answer Key for Vignette 3

Jamie's child-friendly alarm clock starts to play his favorite song when it is time for him to get out of bed. The alarm clock has replaced the need for Taylor to verbally prompt Jamie to get out of bed in the morning. Taylor watches by the doorway to see if Jamie gets up by himself. The song ends and Jamie is still in bed, so she walks to the bed and prompts him to sit up by tapping his shoulder (*partial physical prompt*). Jamie gets out of bed and heads to the bathroom. Taylor goes back to the bedroom doorway but continues to listen to ensure that Jamie is following all the steps of the bathroom routine. Jamie uses the bathroom, steps away before flushing, and turns on the faucet to wash his hands. Taylor steps into the bathroom and points to the flusher on the toilet (*gestural prompt*). Jamie goes back to flush the toilet, and then heads back to the sink to wash his hands. Since the accommodations were put in place with the easier soap pump and the cleared-off vanity, Jamie can now complete the handwashing part of the routine independently. Jamie walks out of the bathroom and toward his clothes. Taylor remains in the bedroom doorway because she knows Jamie is now able to take his pajamas off independently. After taking his pajamas off, Jamie sits on the floor to put on his underwear—only he is about to put them on backwards. Taylor steps in and points to the front of the underwear (*gestural prompt*). Jamie then proceeds to put on his underwear and then his pants. Taylor has asked the physical therapist at school to work with Jamie on putting his pants on without needing to sit on the floor. After putting on his pants, Jamie starts to wander away from the rest of his clothes, so Taylor steps in again and points to his clothes (*gestural prompt*). Although Jamie sometimes still requires prompts to stay on task, the overall number of prompts he needs to complete this part of the morning routine is significantly less than what it had been only a few weeks ago. Taylor knows Jamie still needs some assistance with putting on his shirt, so she stays close by and steps in when needed to guide Jamie's hands to the sleeve holes (*partial physical prompt*). Once his shirt is on, Taylor knows he can independently put on his socks and put his clothes in the hamper, so she heads down the hall toward the top of the stairs. Jamie finishes up his routine and meets Taylor at the top of the stairs. Taylor praises him for doing a great job with this part of his morning routine, gives him his favorite fidget toy, and then they head downstairs for breakfast (*appropriate use of reinforcement*).

Now compare how many of each type of prompt Taylor used during the routine to how many you found, using the following table.

Prompts that Taylor used	How many I found
Full physical prompts—0	
Partial physical prompts—2	
Verbal prompts—0	
Gestural prompts—3	
Model prompts—0	
New positional prompts (the soap is still closer)—0	

Prompts that Taylor used	How many I found
Tasks that Taylor did for Jamie—0	
Total prompts—5	

Now Taylor has gone from 30 prompts to 18 to 5! That's 25 fewer times that she needs to get involved in Jamie's morning routine. Not only is she less exhausted in the morning, but she loves seeing Jamie take the initiative to complete his morning routine on his own. As they have continued to practice, it is also taking Jamie less time to complete his routine, leading to less rushing, more playtime, and just an overall calmer morning altogether.

Now that you understand the basics of prompting, in the next chapter we are going to teach you how to create a task analysis. Having the ability to create and use a task analysis, combined with appropriate use of prompts and prompt fading, will likely change your and your child's day—and hopefully your futures too!

Part IV

Let's Do This!

7

"How Do I Start?"
HOW TO CREATE A TASK ANALYSIS

Gina wanted her daughter Lacey to get herself dressed independently in the morning. The mornings were rushed, and it would be so much easier if she didn't need to stand in Lacey's room and guide her through getting dressed. Lacey knew how to take her clothes off and how to put on her pants and underwear. She needed help to put on her shirt and socks. Lacey seemed to need Gina to guide her to do each step. Gina knew Lacey was capable of putting her clothes in the hamper, but she felt like she needed to remind her every morning or it didn't happen.

One morning after they had walked into Lacey's room, Gina put an outfit out on Lacey's bed, told her to get dressed, and then walked out to the hallway because she wanted to see what Lacey would do if she wasn't in there. Lacey took off her pajamas, leaving them in a pile on the floor. Then she went into her drawer and pulled out a pair of leggings. Gina didn't know if Lacey didn't realize that Gina had left clothes out for her, or didn't want to wear the outfit that she had picked. After putting on the leggings, Lacey took the shirt off the bed. She tried to put it on but could not. Lacey put the shirt back on the bed and started to play with a toy.

One of the most important skills a parent of a neurodiverse child can learn is how to break down a routine into super-small, manageable steps, and then teach those steps to the child. We frequently look at multistep routines as single events. Take, for example, food shopping. It might be listed as one task on our to-do list, despite the fact that it entails a series of smaller tasks, such as creating a shopping list, going to the store, locating those items, paying for them, and bringing them home. We see food shopping as a relatively simple, straightforward, *single* activity—but your child may not.

You know the saying "Success is in the details"? Well, that pearl of wisdom holds true for completing tasks like food shopping, brushing your teeth, showering, getting ready for bed, and making a meal. The inability to complete any of the smaller steps of a multistep routine prevents anyone from completing the routine in its entirety. Most adults take for granted the ease with which we complete daily tasks. However, children who have motor planning delays, muscle weakness, and attention deficits struggle to complete these same tasks. To better understand their experience, think for a moment what your day would look like if your dominant hand was broken and in a cast. All of a sudden, completing these tasks is not so simple anymore. Writing a food shopping list, or even unlocking your phone to dictate the list, becomes a more arduous and time-consuming process. Then, you'd have to figure out an alternative way to get to the market, since driving yourself would not be possible. Being one-handed would have quite an effect on your thoroughness, frustration level, and willingness to complete the activity at all.

Given this perspective, it's likely that your child is having difficulty with one or more microsteps, making their ability to complete the entire routine independently impossible without support. By performing a task analysis, you will be able to better pinpoint which steps your child is having difficulty with. Then, you can either teach your child a new way to complete that step or accommodate them in some way (usually by modifying the environment). By making the routine components more manageable for your child, you set the stage to increase their competence and confidence. Simultaneously, you are also decreasing both their and your frustration level.

From a Single Activity to a Multistep Process

Let's take a look at what a task analysis for food shopping would look like.

EXAMPLE OF A FOOD SHOPPING SEQUENCE

1. Make a food shopping list.
2. Drive to the supermarket.
3. Get a shopping cart.

4. Start in the first section of store that you walk into (usually produce).
5. Collect all the items needed in that section.
6. Move to the next aisle.
7. Collect all the items needed in that aisle.
8. Repeat steps 6 and 7 until you are done shopping.
9. Get in line to check out.
10. Wait your turn in line.
11. Greet the cashier.
12. Unload your items onto the checkout belt.
13. Place your items in bags.
14. Place your bags in your shopping cart.
15. Pay for your items.
16. Thank the cashier.
17. Bring the items to your car.
18. Load the items into your car.
19. Drive home.
20. Unload the items from your car.
21. Unpack the bags and put the food items away.

So, this "simple" activity is really 21 steps! Furthermore, it is quite possible that if you're teaching your child how to food shop for the first time, you would need to break some of these 21 steps down into further microsteps. For example, the first step, "Make food shopping list" is really a multistep process that involves checking what you already have at home, deciding what you need for the upcoming week (or meal), checking the quantity of each item you need and comparing it to how much you currently have, and then writing down what you need to purchase. You may need to take into consideration whether you can get everything in one store or if you will need to go to multiple stores. You also may be shopping on a budget and need to take that into consideration too.

Additionally, there are many decisions that need to be made during food shopping. Do you need a cart, or will a basket be enough? Maybe you don't need either because you are only picking up one or two items. When you arrive in the cereal aisle, maybe the store is out of the cereal you wanted and now you need to pick a different cereal. Or maybe the store has a cereal that you didn't think they would have, and you really want it instead of what you had planned to buy. Do you want to use self-checkout or go to a lane with a cashier? Do you want to use cash, a debit card, or a credit card to pay? Making these decisions is a higher-level skill that you can address once your child learns the fundamentals.

You might be thinking, Well, okay, so food shopping is more involved than I realized, but I just want my child to brush their teeth—that's not so hard! Let's look at the toothbrushing sequence.

1. Walk into the bathroom.
2. Get your toothbrush.
3. Get the toothpaste.
4. Take the cap off the toothpaste.
5. Squeeze an appropriate amount of toothpaste on your toothbrush.
6. Put the cap back on the toothpaste.
7. Turn on the faucet.
8. Wet your toothbrush.
9. Brush the bottom outside of your teeth for 30 seconds.
10. Brush the bottom inside of your teeth for 30 seconds.
11. Brush the top outside of your teeth for 30 seconds.
12. Brush the top inside of your teeth for 30 seconds.
13. Rinse your brush and hands.
14. Rinse your mouth with water.
15. Put your toothbrush away.
16. Wipe off the counter.
17. Dry your hands.
18. Leave the bathroom.

That's 18 steps and it does not even include flossing or using mouthwash! There may not be as many decisions to make with this sequence, but there are a lot of motor demands. Think back to the previous scenario where your dominant hand is in a cast. You might think that is extreme, but the amount of effort and time it would take you to brush your teeth only using your non-dominant hand may be a good representation of how much effort and time your child needs to brush their teeth. This could be because they have motor planning issues, trouble attending, or just because it is a new task for them, and they haven't yet developed the muscle memory to complete it with ease.

We know that it can feel overwhelming to list out all these steps, but the good news is that you only have to do it once for each task you want to target. We aren't expecting you to work on everything at once. In fact, we'd like you to just pick one routine to address at a time. We will guide you through that process later in this chapter. Addressing one thing at a time can help combat any feelings of overwhelm and makes creating a task analysis feel more manageable.

Task Analysis Made Simple

Once you get the hang of task analysis, you can apply this strategy to virtually any multistep task your child needs to complete. We've made creating a task analysis simple for you to do by distilling it into four chronological activities:

1. Documenting the routine
2. Scoring the routine
3. Understanding where and why your child needs help
4. Helping your child

Let's look at each step of the process using toothbrushing as an example.

ACTIVITY: Documenting Your Child's Toothbrushing Sequence

You may have read the 18 steps for toothbrushing and thought, "That's not the way my child brushes his teeth" or "We do things in a different order." That's okay. A task analysis can be customized any way you need or want it to be. For your first activity in this chapter, you are going to make your own sequence to use for a task analysis. While we use the example of toothbrushing, you may feel that your child is not ready to do that by themselves yet or that they are already able to do that independently. If that is the case, choose another routine that you think may be better suited for them; see the "Where Do I Start?" section and the "Choosing a Routine" activity at the end of the chapter.

DIRECTIONS: Set up your camera where it can record the entire routine. Press "record" and pay attention to how your child completes the toothbrushing sequence. Later, play back the recording and take notes, or photocopy or download the Task Analysis Data Worksheet (on the facing page) that you can fill in. Document the individual steps of the sequence in the order that they are completed. Below is a filled-in sample from one parent. Don't worry about scoring yet—we'll cover that next.

Sample Task Analysis with Steps Filled In

Child's name: __John__   Date: __1/15__   Scorer: __Mom__

	Step	Score	Prompt level	Comments
1	Walk into the bathroom	+ −	FP PP G I	
2	Get your toothbrush	+ −	FP PP G I	
3	Get the toothpaste	+ −	FP PP G I	
4	Take the cap off the toothpaste	+ −	FP PP G I	
5	Squeeze an appropriate amount of toothpaste on your toothbrush	+ −	FP PP G I	
6	Put the cap back on the toothpaste	+ −	FP PP G I	
7	Turn on the faucet	+ −	FP PP G I	
8	Wet your toothbrush	+ −	FP PP G I	
9	Brush the bottom outside of your teeth for 30 seconds	+ −	FP PP G I	
10	Brush the bottom inside of your teeth for 30 seconds	+ −	FP PP G I	
11	Brush the top outside of your teeth for 30 seconds	+ −	FP PP G I	
12	Brush the top inside of your teeth for 30 seconds	+ −	FP PP G I	
13	Rinse your toothbrush and hands	+ −	FP PP G I	
14	Rinse your mouth with water	+ −	FP PP G I	
15	Put your toothbrush away	+ −	FP PP G I	
16	Wipe off the counter	+ −	FP PP G I	
17	Dry your hands	+ −	FP PP G I	
18	Leave the bathroom	+ −	FP PP G I	

Task Analysis Data Worksheet

Child's name: _____   Date: _____   Scorer: _____

	Step	Score	Prompt level	Comments
1		+ −	FP PP G I	
2		+ −	FP PP G I	
3		+ −	FP PP G I	
4		+ −	FP PP G I	
5		+ −	FP PP G I	
6		+ −	FP PP G I	
7		+ −	FP PP G I	
8		+ −	FP PP G I	
9		+ −	FP PP G I	
10		+ −	FP PP G I	
11		+ −	FP PP G I	
12		+ −	FP PP G I	
13		+ −	FP PP G I	
14		+ −	FP PP G I	
15		+ −	FP PP G I	
16		+ −	FP PP G I	
17		+ −	FP PP G I	
18		+ −	FP PP G I	
Total + *for each prompt level:*				
Percent + *for each prompt level (total for each prompt level/total number of that prompt)*				

FP = full physical; PP = partial physical; G = gestural; I = independent.

From *Spectrum of Independence* by Kristin Lombardi and Christine Drew. Copyright © 2025 The Guilford Press. Permission to photocopy this material, or to download enlarged printable versions (*www.guilford.com/lombardi-forms*), is granted to purchasers of this book for personal use; see copyright page for details.

TIP: Try to pick a time that is less rushed. For example, if you know that getting your child ready in time for the school bus is a rush every morning, then do this exercise at night. If you have a ton of time in the morning because your child wakes up early and doesn't get picked up until several hours later, feel free to try it then.

ACTIVITY: Scoring the Task Analysis

The next step of the process is to determine which parts of the sequence your child can complete independently (if any), which parts he needs help with, and what that help involves (physical prompt, gestural prompt, model prompt, or positional prompt). In order to determine this, you need to complete a *probe*. During a probe, you see what your child can do without your help. For example, if your goal is for your child to brush their teeth, you set up your recording device, hit record, bring your child to the bathroom, and say, "Brush your teeth." If they don't move forward in the routine for 5–10 seconds, then prompt them through the initial step. Then wait for another 5–10 seconds to see if they will complete the next step. The point of this is to see how much your child will do on their own and not to complete the whole routine for them unnecessarily. Remember, your ultimate goal is for your child to be able to take care of their daily living activities as independently as possible.

DIRECTIONS: Take your personalized list of steps from the activity "Documenting Your Child's Toothbrushing Sequence," and using the information you learned in Chapter 5 about prompting, score each step as your child completes it. You can either watch the video you recorded previously or record a new video. Remember the prompt abbreviations from the prompting chapter: HOH (hand-over-hand)/FP (full physical), PP (partial physical), G (gestural), M (model), P (positional), V (visual), and I (independent). An *independent* response means that you said nothing, did not point at anything, and did not physically guide your child in any way. Basically, any time you do anything that affects the sequence, you are scoring a prompt for that item. You are documenting what you need to do in order to get them through the routine. The only time you should need to circle a minus in the +/− column is if your child is not able to complete a step at the full physical prompt level.

Here is some further guidance:

1. Give your child a chance at each step to complete the step independently (using a brief wait time of 5–10 seconds) before prompting them, as you won't know if there are any steps that they can complete themselves if you automatically prompt them.

2. Note if your child engages in any behaviors that disrupt the sequence, such as leaving the bathroom before he has completed brushing his teeth, resisting prompts, or needing to be redirected back to the task. If at any time you feel your child is struggling to complete a step due to motor planning issues or muscle weakness, note that as well.

3. If they are doing the sequence independently but need you to be standing there supervising, the next step would be to fade your presence gradually (covered in Chapter 8).

4. If they are doing the routine entirely independently, they may be ready to move on to more advanced task analyses like completing their entire morning or evening routine independently.

See the next version of the worksheet on page 138 for an example of a scored task analysis for toothbrushing.

WHY IS MY CHILD NOT COMPLETING A SPECIFIC STEP?

In order to help your child, it is important to understand why they are not completing a specific task in the sequence independently. There are many reasons why a child may not be able to complete a task. We refer to these reasons as independence blockers. It is important to be clear on what those independence blockers are for any step that your child is not able to complete independently. Although it may be tempting to jump ahead to the solutions section, please hold off until you have thoroughly investigated and documented the "why" behind each step that your child is not completing independently. This will lead you to more effective solutions and save you time in the long run.

List of Independence Blockers

- *External events:* Distraction due to external events can take the form of preferred items that direct your child's attention away from their routine

Sample Task Analysis with Scoring Filled In

Child's name: __John__   Date: __1/16__   Scorer: __Mom__

	Step	Score	Prompt level	Comments
1	Walk into the bathroom	⊕ –	FP PP G Ⓘ	
2	Get your toothbrush	⊕ –	FP PP G Ⓘ	
3	Get the toothpaste	⊕ –	FP PP G Ⓘ	
4	Take the cap off the toothpaste	⊕ –	FP ⓅⓅ G I	
5	Squeeze an appropriate amount of toothpaste on your toothbrush	+ ⊖	ⒻⓅ PP G I	Child resisted prompt
6	Put the cap back on the toothpaste	⊕ –	FP ⓅⓅ G I	
7	Turn on the faucet	⊕ –	FP PP G Ⓘ	
8	Wet your toothbrush	⊕ –	FP PP G Ⓘ	
9	Brush the bottom outside of your teeth for 30 seconds	⊕ –	ⒻⓅ PP G I	
10	Brush the bottom inside of your teeth for 30 seconds	⊕ –	ⒻⓅ PP G I	
11	Brush the top outside of your teeth for 30 seconds	+ ⊖	ⒻⓅ PP G I	Child resisted prompt
12	Brush the top inside of your teeth for 30 seconds	+ ⊖	ⒻⓅ PP G I	Child resisted prompt
13	Rinse your brush and hands	⊕ –	FP PP G Ⓘ	
14	Rinse your mouth with water	⊕ –	FP ⓅⓅ G I	
15	Put your toothbrush away	⊕ –	FP PP Ⓖ I	
16	Wipe off the counter	⊕ –	ⒻⓅ PP G I	
17	Dry your hands	⊕ –	FP ⓅⓅ G I	
18	Leave the bathroom	⊕ –	FP PP G Ⓘ	
Total + for each prompt level:			3 4 1 7	
Percent + for each prompt level (total for each prompt level/total number of that prompt)			50 100 100 100	

FP = full physical; PP = partial physical; G = gestural; I = independent.

(toys, television, books, and so on), as well as aversive sounds that upset your child and create an environment that is not conducive to focusing (running the vacuum or hair dryer if your child is sensitive to noise, background noise from your other children or animals in the household).

- *Internal events:* A child can be distracted by internal events such as stereotypic behavior, fixations on a specific topic, or feelings of distress or frustration.

- *Motor planning:* Difficulty with motor planning, or the body's ability to organize movements in order to do a task, can affect a child's ability to complete certain motor tasks. For example, your child places their hands on the ladder to the slide but has trouble coordinating their feet to climb.

- *Muscle weakness:* Lack of muscular strength can make completing certain activities very challenging, especially those that require balance (putting on pants or socks while standing), hand strength (opening or closing containers, cutting food with a knife, grasping socks), or heavy lifting (putting a large container of toys on a shelf, unpacking bulky or heavy grocery items).

- *Inappropriate environment arrangements:* Environmental arrangements can play a big role in your child's level of independence. Some common examples of inappropriate environmental arrangements include having needed items out of reach (towels, clothes), having developmentally inappropriate items that your child can't maneuver (a glass soap dispenser, tight clothes), a messy or cluttered environment (this makes it very hard for a child to stay organized), and not keeping items in a specified place (this creates a situation where your child needs to look for the needed items each time they engage in the routine).

- *Developmentally inappropriate expectations:* For this block, you want to determine if you are asking your child to complete a task that is within their reach developmentally. For example, if your child can't put on their pants independently or pour an appropriate amount of cereal into a bowl, it would be unfair to expect them to get ready for school independently each morning.

- *Lack of appropriate consequences—escape:* This block can be particularly challenging if you have a history of not following through with your directives. Telling your child to do something and then letting them get away with not completing the task leads to your child learning that they can ignore you. Getting away with not completing a task includes both allowing the task to not be completed at all as well as you doing the task for them.

- *Lack of appropriate consequences—no reinforcer:* For this blocker, we need to be mindful of creating a situation where there is some meaningful reason from your child's perspective to complete the routine that you need them to complete. For example, you might feel that having fresh breath after you brush your teeth is enough reason for you to brush them. Your child may not feel the same. If your child does not enjoy brushing his teeth, and then you have him go to bed after brushing his teeth when you know that he hates going to bed, you have a nonpreferred task followed by another nonpreferred task. Instead, try to provide a reinforcing activity once he completes a nonpreferred task. This could mean starting the toothbrushing routine 15 minutes earlier, and then having your child play for 15 minutes before bed as their reinforcer.

- *Unintentional reinforcement:* Sometimes we create situations where we provide access to preferred activities when we don't mean to—for example, letting your child watch television (if that is a highly preferred activity) while they are supposed to be getting dressed (not a highly preferred activity). In this scenario, you want them to focus on getting dressed before giving them access to the television.

- *Repeated practice of inappropriate behavior within the sequence:* A common example of this is every time your child turns the water on in the sink, they start playing with the water instead of brushing their teeth. Now this behavior has become part of the routine—in essence, a habit. In these cases, you want to use errorless teaching. Errorless teaching is a teaching method where you prompt your child before they have the chance to make a mistake and direct them back to the task before they have a chance to engage in the inappropriate behavior.

- *Difficulty breaking a situational routine:* Sometimes children with developmental or intellectual disabilities may be rigid when it comes to switching up known routines. For example, you have been letting them eat dinner in the playroom while they watch a show, and now have decided that they need to eat dinner without a show playing. Your child has a tantrum because they are in the playroom with their dinner and looking for you to put on their show. If your child is having trouble changing a routine due to resistance to change, sometimes making a big change can make things easier. For example, in this scenario, it may be easier to switch dinner to the kitchen because that location is not associated with watching a show.

Each of these reasons has specific remedies that can be applied to move past the challenge and allow the child to complete the task independently. In order to do that, you need to break the task down, pinpoint which steps are not able to be done independently, and then determine why each step can't be completed before determining the remedy. This leads us to our next activity.

ACTIVITY: Understanding "Why" Your Child Needs Help

PREPARATION: Look back over your scored task analysis as you watch the video again. You will find that for this step in particular, having a video to analyze will be much easier than trying to do this in the moment. As you watch the sequence unfold, make a note as to why you think you needed to get involved for each step you scored as a prompt. Use the list of independence blockers as guidance and add your own reasons if needed. You will use this information to complete Activities 1 and 2.

ACTIVITY 1: HELPING MY CHILD

Now that you have gathered all this information, you are ready to start teaching your child so they will be able to eventually complete the sequence on their own. This activity is broken down into three parts: assess the environment, assess your child's behavior, and gradually teach independence.

Assess the Environment

The first thing you want to do is address any environmental issues that may be inhibiting your child's independence. Environmental issues can lead to distractions or create a situation where your child is unnecessarily struggling to complete a task that they would otherwise be able to complete. There are several steps you can take to address these issues.

First, a child may have difficulty breaking a situational routine. For example, your child may be used to going into a specific bathroom and having you brush his teeth while he is taking a bath. Now you are asking him to go into the same bathroom and brush his own teeth before he gets into the bath. Due to his adherence to routines, he is having trouble breaking his known routine and engaging in the new routine you want him to engage in.

Sample Task Analysis for a Child with Motor Planning Challenges

Child's name: __John__   Date: __1/17__   Scorer: __Mom__

	Step	Score	Prompt level	Comments
1	Walk into the bathroom	⊕ −	FP PP G Ⓘ	
2	Get your toothbrush	⊕ −	FP PP G Ⓘ	
3	Get the toothpaste	⊕ −	FP PP G Ⓘ	
4	Take the cap off the toothpaste	⊕ −	FP ⓅⓅ G I	Motor planning
5	Squeeze an appropriate amount of toothpaste on your toothbrush	+ ⊖	ⒻⓅ PP G I	Resisted prompt
6	Put the cap back on the toothpaste	⊕ −	FP ⓅⓅ G I	Motor planning
7	Turn on the faucet	⊕ −	FP PP G Ⓘ	
8	Wet your toothbrush	⊕ −	FP PP G Ⓘ	
9	Brush the bottom outside of your teeth for 30 seconds	⊕ −	ⒻⓅ PP G I	Motor planning, used to having me do it for him
10	Brush the bottom inside of your teeth for 30 seconds	⊕ −	ⒻⓅ PP G I	Motor planning, used to having me do it for him
11	Brush the top outside of your teeth for 30 seconds	+ ⊖	ⒻⓅ PP G I	Resisted prompt
12	Brush the top inside of your teeth for 30 seconds	+ ⊖	ⒻⓅ PP G I	Resisted prompt
13	Rinse your brush and hands	⊕ −	FP PP G Ⓘ	
14	Rinse your mouth with water	+ ⊖	FP ⓅⓅ G I	Refused to do this even with guidance
15	Put your toothbrush away	⊕ −	FP PP Ⓖ I	Child became distracted and needed to be redirected
16	Wipe off the counter	⊕ −	ⒻⓅ PP G I	Child tried to leave bathroom to get iPad
17	Dry your hands	⊕ −	FP ⓅⓅ G I	Prompt for thoroughness due to motor planning
18	Leave the bathroom	⊕ −	FP PP G Ⓘ	
	Total + for each prompt level:		3 3 1 7	
	Percent + for each prompt level (total for each prompt level/total number of that prompt)		50 75 100 100	

FP = full physical; PP = partial physical; G = gestural; I = independent.

Sample Task Analysis for a Child Whose Primary Barrier Is the Environment

Child's name: __Lucy__ Date: __3/21__ Scorer: __Dad__

	Step	Score	Prompt level	Comments
1	Walk into the bathroom	(+) −	FP PP G (I)	
2	Get your toothbrush	(+) −	FP PP G (I)	
3	Get the toothpaste	(+) −	FP PP G (I)	
4	Take the cap off the toothpaste	(+) −	FP (PP) G I	She couldn't reach the toothpaste
5	Squeeze an appropriate amount of toothpaste on your toothbrush	+ (−)	(FP) PP G I	The container was empty
6	Put the cap back on the toothpaste	(+) −	FP (PP) G I	She couldn't find the cap because it rolled behind toys on the counter
7	Turn on the faucet	(+) −	FP PP G (I)	
8	Wet your toothbrush	(+) −	FP PP G (I)	
9	Brush the bottom outside of your teeth for 30 seconds	(+) −	(FP) PP G I	Her favorite part of a movie came on his iPad (which she brought into the bathroom) and she was distracted
10	Brush the bottom inside of your teeth for 30 seconds	+ (−)	(FP) PP G I	Since I started brushing, I just finished it for her
11	Brush the top outside of your teeth for 30 seconds	+ (−)	(FP) PP G I	Since I started brushing, I just finished it for her
12	Brush the top inside of your teeth for 30 seconds	+ (−)	(FP) PP G I	Since I started brushing, I just finished it for her
13	Rinse your brush and hands	(+) −	FP PP G (I)	
14	Rinse your mouth with water	(+) −	FP (PP) G I	She got distracted by an empty box on the counter and when I removed it she wanted to tell me about star constellations
15	Put your toothbrush away	(+) −	FP PP (G) I	She tried but the toothbrush holder was full
16	Wipe off the counter	(+) −	(FP) PP G I	There were no paper towels to wipe the counter
17	Dry your hands	(+) −	(FP) PP G I	She can't reach the towel
18	Leave the bathroom	(+) −	FP PP G (I)	
	Total + for each prompt level:		2 3 1 7	
	Percent + for each prompt level (total for each prompt level/total number of that prompt)		29 100 100 100	

FP = full physical; PP = partial physical; G = gestural; I = independent.

In these cases, sometimes making a big change, like switching which bathroom you use to teach him to brush his teeth, or switching up the order of events can help reset the routine.

Second, modify the environment to decrease the potential for distraction. Using the toothbrushing sequence as an example, remove any toys or other unnecessary items from the bathroom that your child may be tempted to play with instead of brushing his teeth. Also, make sure your child is not bringing toys or electronics into the bathroom with them. If they were in the middle of playing with something before you asked them to brush their teeth, it will be right where they left it, and they can return to it as soon as they are finished.

Next, modify the environment to make it accessible to your child. Make sure your child can reach his toothbrush, the toothpaste, the faucet handles, and a towel. Make sure there is toothpaste in the tube of toothpaste. Rolling the end of the toothpaste tube down as you use it and clipping it with a binder clip can be a big help. You can also get the specialized dispensers that do not have a cap and automatically pump the toothpaste onto the toothbrush based on sensors. If your child can't access something he needs to complete the sequence, this will be an immediate independence blocker.

Finally, make any general modifications that will make the task less aversive and easier overall. For example, try to choose a toothpaste flavor that your child likes. Regulate the water temperature in your home so the water does not get scalding hot. If your child will tolerate it, try an electric toothbrush with a built-in timer—these brushes beep every 30 seconds to let you know to move to the next quarter of your mouth.

If you needed to make a lot of modifications, record the routine again and then rescore the task analysis the next time your child brushes their teeth. You may find that they are able to do more steps independently than you initially scored.

Assess Your Child's Behavior

The next step is to address any problem behavior that may be occurring. If your child is leaving the bathroom before brushing his teeth, refusing to brush his teeth, waiting for you to brush his teeth for him, whining, explaining to you why he shouldn't have to brush his teeth, or delaying brushing his teeth (meaning you have to ask him multiple times before he will stop what he is doing and go brush his teeth), you are going to want to refer back to Chapter 4 and look at the following items:

- Are you being clear in your directives? Example: Are you saying something like, "Well, it's almost time to leave the house, so we better get ready. Your teeth haven't been brushed yet . . . " or are you stating "John, it is time to brush your teeth"?

- Are you following through with your directives? Example: If John does not stop what he is doing and head to the bathroom, are you stopping what you are doing to guide him to the bathroom? How long do you allow him to delay starting the task?

- Are you applying appropriate and consistent consequences? Example: Have you told John that he can watch a TV show only after he brushes his teeth? Or has John already done everything he wanted to do and now the only consequence to brushing his teeth is going to bed? Think about it this way: If he hates going to bed, you are in essence punishing him for brushing his teeth.

Gradually Teach Independence

Once you have addressed any environmental issues and established instructional control (your child is following directions and understands what the consequences are for brushing or not brushing his teeth), you are ready to start teaching your child how to increase their independence during the routine. You will do this in three ways:

- Be mindful of your involvement: We know it is faster and easier in the moment to jump in and either prompt your child or do it for them, but in the long run, you will both be better off if you give your child the time, space, and encouragement he needs to complete tasks on his own.

- Practice, practice, practice! Kids with motor planning delays need a lot of practice. Often, they are able to learn to do things independently, they just need more repetitions of practice then a child who does not have a delay. This can also be a time when working with an occupational therapist may be helpful.

- Systematically fade your prompts: Refer to Chapter 8.

ACTIVITY 2: TROUBLESHOOTING WORKSHEET

If your child is struggling with a routine, use the Troubleshooting Worksheet on the facing page to ensure that you have taken all the steps to remove barriers and facilitate the routine.

My Child Can't (or Won't) Do Any of the Steps! Forward and Backward Chaining

We frequently ask parents, "What would happen if you left your child alone in their bedroom and told them to get dressed? Would they get dressed?" The answer we get is usually "No," followed by many variations of the child engaging in off-task behavior, whether playing, going back to bed, engaging in stereotypic behavior, or flat-out leaving the room still in their pajamas to go find Mommy. So far in this chapter, we have been discussing what's known as *total task chaining*. If your child is not making progress using this, you may want to try forward or backward chaining.

Forward chaining is a teaching procedure where the parent prompts the child to do the first step in the sequence and then the parent completes the rest of the steps for them. For example, to forward chain the toothbrushing sequence, your first step would be to physically prompt your child to walk into the bathroom. You then have a choice; you could complete the rest of the routine for your child or prompt them to finish the routine. This depends on the routine you've chosen and what works best for your child. Then you would fade your prompts until your child was independently walking into the bathroom. Once they are walking to the bathroom independently, you would start by physically prompting your child to complete the next step of the routine, which would be to get out their toothbrush.

Then you would fade that prompt as well, by working down the prompting hierarchy (full physical to partial physical to model or gesture to independence). Once your child is able to complete the first and second steps independently, continue the process of

Troubleshooting Worksheet

Have I...	Yes	No
Determined that this task is developmentally appropriate?		
Removed distractions in the environment? (e.g., electronics, toys)		
Ensured that all the materials needed for the routine are accessible to my child? (e.g., towel is within their reach, toothpaste is on bathroom vanity)		
Ensured that all aspects of the routine are physically accessible to my child? (e.g., replaced snap-on pants with pull-on pants, glass soap jar with plastic soap pump)		
Set up the routine to be tolerable to my child? (e.g., bought toothpaste that they like, bought clothes that are comfortable for them)		
Checked for past routines that may have turned into hard-to-break habits?		
Clearly stated what I am expecting my child to do? (e.g., "It's time to put away your toys and take a shower" instead of "Are you ready to take a shower?")		
Followed through with my directives?		
Reinforced appropriate behavior?		
Redirected inappropriate behavior?		
Provided consistent and timely consequences following appropriate and inappropriate behavior?		
Pinpointed the exact steps within the sequence that are challenging for my child?		
Increased the prompt level for the steps that are difficult?		
Assessed if my child is motivated to complete the routine? (i.e., whether innately or due to external reinforcement)		

From *Spectrum of Independence* by Kristin Lombardi and Christine Drew. Copyright © 2025 The Guilford Press. Permission to photocopy this material, or to download enlarged printable versions (*www.guilford.com/lombardi-forms*), is granted to purchasers of this book for personal use; see copyright page for details.

teaching each step in sequence: (See the worksheets on pages 149 and 150.) While this process may take longer, this may be necessary for some children.

Now for backward chaining. Backward chaining is the reverse of forward chaining—the parent completes all the steps of a task for their child except for the final step. Then prompt your child to complete the last step. Then you will fade those prompts until your child is independently completing that step. Next you would begin to prompt the second to last step of the routine and then fade that prompt as well. The nice part about backward chaining is that the reinforcer of completing the last step in the sequence—in this case, putting their toothbrush away independently—can be easily followed by play time. In another example, completing the last step of making a smoothie is naturally followed by getting to drink it. We all love a quick payout! For examples of backward chaining, see the worksheets on pages 151 and 152.

What To Do if Your Child Is Struggling

There are myriad reasons that your child may not complete a sequence independently. As frustrating as this may be, the good news is that in the vast majority of cases, there's an effective solution that comes from taking a closer look at the situation. It takes persistence and patience, but by looking at the situation from many angles, you can often locate the problem that was lying just outside your awareness.

As an example, let's look at several reasons why a child is not completing the toothbrushing sequence independently, as well as the recommended solution to each scenario.

- Inability to stay on task due to external distractions
  - Provide a strong reinforcer at the end of the routine
  - Complete a probe using a visual schedule (either picture or words)
  - Limit distractions in the environment, such as turning off the television or putting away preferred toys

Sample Task Analysis of Forward Chaining, First Step

Child's name: __Andrew__   Date: __2/20__   Scorer: __Mom__

	Step	Score	Prompt level	Comments
1	Walk into the bathroom	+ −	FP PP G I	Begin by fading prompts for this step.
2	Get your toothbrush	+ −	FP PP G I	Parent completes the remaining steps.
3	Get the toothpaste	+ −	FP PP G I	Parent completes.
4	Take the cap off the toothpaste	+ −	FP PP G I	Parent completes.
5	Squeeze an appropriate amount of toothpaste on your toothbrush	+ −	FP PP G I	Parent completes.
6	Put the cap back on the toothpaste	+ −	FP PP G I	Parent completes.
7	Turn on the faucet	+ −	FP PP G I	Parent completes.
8	Wet your toothbrush	+ −	FP PP G I	Parent completes.
9	Brush the bottom outside of your teeth for 30 seconds	+ −	FP PP G I	Parent completes.
10	Brush the bottom inside of your teeth for 30 seconds	+ −	FP PP G I	Parent completes.
11	Brush the top outside of your teeth for 30 seconds	+ −	FP PP G I	Parent completes.
12	Brush the top inside of your teeth for 30 seconds	+ −	FP PP G I	Parent completes.
13	Rinse your brush and hands	+ −	FP PP G I	Parent completes.
14	Rinse your mouth with water	+ −	FP PP G I	Parent completes.
15	Put your toothbrush away	+ −	FP PP G I	Parent completes.
16	Wipe off the counter	+ −	FP PP G I	Parent completes.
17	Dry your hands	+ −	FP PP G I	Parent completes.
18	Leave the bathroom	+ −	FP PP G I	Parent completes.

Sample Task Analysis of Forward Chaining, Second Step

Child's name: __Andrew__   Date: __3/1__   Scorer: __Mom__

	Step	Score	Prompt level	Comments
1	Walk into the bathroom	(+) −	FP PP G (I)	Ind.
2	Get your toothbrush	(+) −	FP (PP) G I	Parent completes the remaining steps.
3	Get the toothpaste	+ −	FP PP G I	Parent completes.
4	Take the cap off the toothpaste	+ −	FP PP G I	Parent completes.
5	Squeeze an appropriate amount of toothpaste on your toothbrush	+ −	FP PP G I	Parent completes.
6	Put the cap back on the toothpaste	+ −	FP PP G I	Parent completes.
7	Turn on the faucet	+ −	FP PP G I	Parent completes.
8	Wet your toothbrush	+ −	FP PP G I	Parent completes.
9	Brush the bottom outside of your teeth for 30 seconds	+ −	FP PP G I	Parent completes.
10	Brush the bottom inside of your teeth for 30 seconds	+ −	FP PP G I	Parent completes.
11	Brush the top outside of your teeth for 30 seconds	+ −	FP PP G I	Parent completes.
12	Brush the top inside of your teeth for 30 seconds	+ −	FP PP G I	Parent completes.
13	Rinse your brush and hands	+ −	FP PP G I	Parent completes.
14	Rinse your mouth with water	+ −	FP PP G I	Parent completes.
15	Put your toothbrush away	+ −	FP PP G I	Parent completes.
16	Wipe off the counter	+ −	FP PP G I	Parent completes.
17	Dry your hands	+ −	FP PP G I	Parent completes.
18	Leave the bathroom	+ −	FP PP G I	Parent completes.

Sample Task Analysis of Backward Chaining, First Step

Child's name: __Donavon__   Date: __10/8__   Scorer: __Dad__

	Step	Score	Prompt level	Comments
1	Walk into the bathroom	+ −	FP PP G I	Parent completes.
2	Get your toothbrush	+ −	FP PP G I	Parent completes.
3	Get the toothpaste	+ −	FP PP G I	Parent completes.
4	Take the cap off the toothpaste	+ −	FP PP G I	Parent completes.
5	Squeeze an appropriate amount of toothpaste on your toothbrush	+ −	FP PP G I	Parent completes.
6	Put the cap back on the toothpaste	+ −	FP PP G I	Parent completes.
7	Turn on the faucet	+ −	FP PP G I	Parent completes.
8	Wet your toothbrush	+ −	FP PP G I	Parent completes.
9	Brush the bottom outside of your teeth for 30 seconds	+ −	FP PP G I	Parent completes.
10	Brush the bottom inside of your teeth for 30 seconds	+ −	FP PP G I	Parent completes.
11	Brush the top outside of your teeth for 30 seconds	+ −	FP PP G I	Parent completes.
12	Brush the top inside of your teeth for 30 seconds	+ −	FP PP G I	Parent completes.
13	Rinse your brush and hands	+ −	FP PP G I	Parent completes.
14	Rinse your mouth with water	+ −	FP PP G I	Parent completes.
15	Put your toothbrush away	+ −	FP PP G I	Parent completes.
16	Wipe off the counter	+ −	FP PP G I	Parent completes.
17	Dry your hands	+ −	FP PP G I	Parent completes.
18	Leave the bathroom	+ −	FP PP G I	Fade prompts to independent.

Sample Task Analysis of Backward Chaining, Second Step

Child's name: **Donavon**   Date: **10/15**   Scorer: **Dad**

	Step	Score	Prompt level	Comments
1	Walk into the bathroom	+ −	FP PP G I	Parent completes.
2	Get your toothbrush	+ −	FP PP G I	Parent completes.
3	Get the toothpaste	+ −	FP PP G I	Parent completes.
4	Take the cap off the toothpaste	+ −	FP PP G I	Parent completes.
5	Squeeze an appropriate amount of toothpaste on your toothbrush	+ −	FP PP G I	Parent completes.
6	Put the cap back on the toothpaste	+ −	FP PP G I	Parent completes.
7	Turn on the faucet	+ −	FP PP G I	Parent completes.
8	Wet your toothbrush	+ −	FP PP G I	Parent completes.
9	Brush the bottom outside of your teeth for 30 seconds	+ −	FP PP G I	Parent completes.
10	Brush the bottom inside of your teeth for 30 seconds	+ −	FP PP G I	Parent completes.
11	Brush the top outside of your teeth for 30 seconds	+ −	FP PP G I	Parent completes.
12	Brush the top inside of your teeth for 30 seconds	+ −	FP PP G I	Parent completes.
13	Rinse your brush and hands	+ −	FP PP G I	Parent completes.
14	Rinse your mouth with water	+ −	FP PP G I	Parent completes.
15	Put your toothbrush away	+ −	FP PP G I	Parent completes.
16	Wipe off the counter	+ −	FP PP G I	Parent completes.
17	Dry your hands	+ −	(FP) PP G I	Fade prompts to independent.
18	Leave the bathroom	+ −	FP PP G (I)	

- Inability to stay on task due to internal distractions
    - Provide strong reinforcement for on-task behavior and completing the whole task
    - Redirect your child using gestural prompts to interrupt any stereotypic behavior
    - Fade your presence incrementally
- Motor planning or muscle weakness
    - Enlist the help of an occupational therapist or physical therapist
    - Accommodate the child by making both the environment and the items in it accessible to them—for example, putting things that they need to complete the routine in reach or grouped together to ease access, purchasing items like soap and shampoo dispensers that they can manipulate, and making sure their clothes have a little bit of wiggle room so they can easily dress themselves
    - Practice. Sometimes children with motor planning delays just need more practice than children without motor planning delays; repetition can be the answer.
- Ineffective environment arrangement
    - Confirm your child can reach everything they need to complete the task—things like a stool to reach the sink or a lower coat hook for their jacket can be really helpful.
    - Ensure the routine is as pleasant as possible for your child—using a child-sized toothbrush, kid-flavored toothpaste, easy-dispensing toothpaste, or a favorite character-themed toothbrush can make the routine that much more enjoyable.
    - Confirm you are providing your child with age-appropriate or developmentally appropriate equipment to the best of your ability—for example, having a plastic soap dispenser in the bathroom instead of a glass one, buying your child a toothbrush with a thicker handle that is easier for them to grasp, or placing a hook for them to hang their coat at a height that they can reach can make completing a task more accessible.
    - Eliminate unnecessary distractions in the environment—putting toys away, turning the TV off, and making sure your phone is silenced are all ways to decrease the distractions in the environment and help your child be successful.

- Inappropriate developmental expectations
  - Every child develops at a different rate. Check with any of the professionals that work directly with your child (pediatricians, teachers, therapists) to see if what you are asking your child to do is appropriate given their current developmental stage.
- Lack of motivation to complete the task independently
  - Provide strong reinforcement at the end of the routine.
  - Fade the parent's presence incrementally.

If your child is not engaging in any part of the task independently, you need to figure out why. First, are they able to complete the smaller tasks motorically? If a child can't put on his pants independently, there is no way he will be able to complete the larger task sequence of getting himself dressed in the morning. The first step would be to teach your child to put each article of clothing on independently, and then move to teaching the sequence of getting dressed. If the child can put his clothes on in terms of motor skills, but can't get through the entire sequence of dressing themselves unless you are providing a constant stream of verbal redirection, then that's a different issue altogether. In the latter case, you would focus on finding the appropriate reinforcer, create a plan to fade your prompts, and then fade yourself from the room.

Where Do I Start?

Picking the correct routine to start with is an important first step. We recommend you choose from a list of daily activities and routines that your child needs to complete, which we walk you through in the "Choosing a Routine" activity below. This way, you are creating a task analysis of something your child is doing every day. One child might be working on getting themselves dressed independently, while another may be working on completing their entire morning routine independently. A child could be in charge of caring for an animal as part of their family chores. One child may need to travel back and forth between parents' houses, so packing a bag could be an important routine. These are just a few of the routines that children may need to master to live more independently in your home. Rather than relying on assessments to tell you what routines and skills to target, we would like you to target the routines that mean the most to you and your child.

ACTIVITY: Choosing a Routine

1. Document each routine your child completes either daily (getting up, getting dressed, putting on pj's, getting ready for meals, handwashing) or five days a week (after-school routine, packing lunch for school). Break down the routine that you choose as far as you need to. For example, "getting ready for school" is probably too big. Within "getting ready for school" you have hygiene, dressing, toileting, eating a meal, and maybe even more. Refer to the list below and on the next page for ideas and places to start.

2. Take the list and underline the routines that have no pressing time limit (toothbrushing at night, putting on pj's, eating dinner).

3. Of your underlined routines, circle the routine that you feel your child is closest to attaining independently.

4. If you still have more than one option, pick the one that will have the greatest effect on your and your child's day to day life. This is your optimal routine to start with.

5. Once you have decided which routine to target, return to the section titled "Task Analysis Made Simple" starting on page 133 and proceed through the process of creating a task analysis.

Here's why: Daily routines are first because your child will use this routine consistently, will get more practice opportunities, and is more likely to retain the routine. The reason we want the one they're doing best on is so that we can capitalize on the success they're already experiencing and we're closer to the finish line. We want your child to experience some early success. We want you to feel the success too. Getting yourself out of the dressing routine may be your first priority because it makes it hard for you to help your other children during bedtime. That's a powerful motivator for you. Now that you have set you and your child up for success by choosing an appropriate routine to target, continue forward into the rest of this chapter.

Here's an example of what the list might look like once you finish:

Get up   Toileting
Take off pj's   Playtime
Put on clothes (school uniform)   Homework

Eat breakfast   Get ready for therapy session
Wash hands   Therapy
Pack lunch   Dinner
Pack backpack   Bath/shower
Put on shoes   (Brush teeth)
Get on bus   (Put on pj's)
Put backpack and lunch away   Bedtime routine
Change from school uniform to afternoon clothes

Some families have difficulty deciding what routines their child should be independent with based on their developmental stage and chronological age. The goal is for your child to be as independent as possible, but what we really need to ask is this: What is your child capable of developmentally, and would we expect a typically developing peer of the same age to be completing this task independently? For example, we would not expect a two-year-old to be potty trained, but it would be appropriate to expect a five-year-old to be. We would not expect a four-year-old to make their own breakfast, but it would be an appropriate expectation for a 12-year-old to make their own bowl of cereal. Keeping your child's age and developmental level in mind will help you choose the right routine for your child. Choosing the right routine will help move your child toward greater independence. Consider the lists below a starting point for routines that may be included in your child's day.

List of Daily Independent Living Skills

Wake up to alarm   Prepare basic meals/snacks
Dress themselves   Pack lunch
Put dirty clothes in laundry   Pack backpack
Use the bathroom/toilet   After school (change clothes, wash
Wash hands   hands, eat snack)
Bathe/shower   Put on pj's
Brush/fix hair   Bedtime routine (brush teeth, read
Wash face   stories, sing songs)
Make bed   Feed and give water to pet
Brush teeth   Pick up toys
Meals (set the table, serve food,   Participate in religious practice
    eat, put plates in sink, wash safe
    dishes, pour drinks)

List of Weekly Independent Living Skills

Laundry (fold and put away clothes, put clothes in washer, put clothes in dryer)
Water plants
Put groceries away
Sweep and use a dustpan

Take out trash
Change bedsheets
Vacuum
Dust

Sequences for Other Everyday Tasks

Just like you, your child is faced with numerous tasks to get through each day. Remember that activities we may consider simple and rote can seem monumental for a neurodiverse child—but that doesn't mean they are impossible. Using the process of task analysis, you can break down a chore into microsteps and gradually teach them to complete the task independently.

Here are a few other examples of task analyses:

SHOWERING

1. Pick out or grab clothes or pajamas you are changing into
2. Bring clothes into bathroom and place on vanity
3. Close the door
4. Get towel and washcloth
5. Take off clothes
6. Turn on water
7. Manage/select water temperature
8. Get in shower
9. Close shower door or curtain behind you
10. Wet your body
11. Wet your hair
12. Use soap and washcloth to wash your body (can be broken down further into separate task analysis)
13. Rinse your body
14. Wring out washcloth and hang to dry
15. Use shampoo to wash your hair (can be broken down further into separate task analysis—see the next page)
16. Rinse your hair
17. Use conditioner in your hair (can be broken down further into separate task analysis)

18. Rinse your hair
19. Turn the shower off
20. Get towel
21. Dry body
22. Put on lotion
23. Get dressed
24. Hang towel
25. Put dirty clothes in the hamper

WASHING HAIR

1. Wet hair
2. Identify which bottle is the shampoo
3. Pick up shampoo bottle
4. Open the bottle
5. Put a small amount of shampoo in your hand
6. Close the bottle
7. Lather the shampoo in your hair
8. Rinse the shampoo out of your hair
9. Identify the conditioner bottle
10. Open the conditioner bottle
11. Put a small amount of conditioner in your hand
12. Close the bottle
13. Rub the conditioner into your hair
14. Wait 1 minute
15. Rinse the conditioner from your hair

As you can see, showering is 25 steps, but here we added another 15 steps just for washing and conditioning your hair. And a child with a developmental delay can get caught up in any one of these steps for a variety of reasons, including identifying which bottle is the shampoo if they can't read, opening the bottle if they have motor issues, or staying on task until the activity is done if they have attention issues.

MAKING LUNCH FOR SCHOOL

1. Get lunch box (microsteps could be: walk to cabinet, open cabinet, identify lunch box, grab lunch box, bring lunch box to kitchen counter)
2. Get water bottle

3. Get ice pack from freezer
4. Put ice pack in lunch box
5. Fill water bottle with water (could be broken down into unscrew lid, go to refrigerator door, press button on refrigerator to select water, place bottle under spout, press bottle back to activate water, watch for when the bottle is nearing full, move bottle away from spout to stop water, screw lid on)
6. Put water bottle in lunch box
7. Put juice box in lunch box
8. Put 1 pack of crackers in lunch box
9. Get 2 cheese wheels from fridge and put in lunch box
10. Get container of cut-up fruit from fridge and put in lunch box
11. Close lunch box
12. Put lunch box in backpack

Activities of Daily Living Examples

HYGIENE

- Washing hands
- Washing face
- Showering
- Brushing teeth
- Brushing hair
- Putting on deodorant
- Cleaning nails
- Using mouthwash and floss

DRESSING

- Dressing and undressing self (underwear, pants, shirt, socks, hat)
- Putting on and taking off shoes
- Tying and untying shoes
- Buckling fastenings (buttons, snaps, buckles)
- Putting on and taking off a jacket
- Zipping and unzipping a jacket
- Completing the entire dressing sequence independently
- Choosing appropriate clothing given the weather and/or activity
- Putting dirty clothes in the hamper

HOME LIVING SKILLS

- Getting a snack
- Packing lunch for school
- Preparing a simple meal for breakfast, lunch, or dinner at home (frozen waffles, sandwich, chicken nuggets)
- Setting and clearing the table
- Emptying and loading the dishwasher
- Keeping bedroom/playroom organized

Examples of How to Break Those Activities Down

Each one of the activities just listed can be broken down in multiple steps. Here are a few examples.

WASHING HANDS

1. Turn on water to correct temperature
2. Wet hands
3. Get soap
4. Pump soap into hand or lather using bar soap
5. Put soap back (if using bar soap)
6. Lather soap on hands for at least 20 seconds
7. Rinse hands
8. Turn off water
9. Get towel
10. Dry hands
11. Put towel back on bar

BRUSHING HAIR

1. Get brush
2. Brush right side
3. Brush left side
4. Brush down the back (middle)
5. Check quality in mirror
6. Brush any messy parts again
7. Put brush away

TAKING OFF SHOES

1. Sit down on floor or in chair
2. Untie shoes (this is important if you want to eventually teach your child how to tie their shoes)
3. Put right hand on left heel and push shoe off
4. Repeat with left hand and right heel
5. Pick up shoes
6. Put shoes away

ZIPPING JACKET

1. Take left side of jacket in left hand (on bottom where zipper starts)
2. Take right side of jacket in right hand (on bottom where zipper starts)
3. Make sure zipper is all the way down to bottom of jacket
4. Insert thin part of zipper into the zipper
5. Pull zipper up

MAKING A BOWL OF CEREAL

1. Get bowl
2. Get spoon
3. Get napkin
4. Get milk
5. Get cereal
6. Open cereal container
7. Pour cereal into bowl
8. Close cereal container
9. Remove milk cap
10. Pour milk into cereal
11. Place cap back on milk
12. Put milk back in fridge
13. Eat cereal
14. Put cereal away when finished eating
15. Put bowl and spoon in the sink
16. Put napkin in the garbage
17. Wipe off the table

SETTING THE TABLE

1. Find out how many people are eating dinner
2. Count out needed plates
3. Count out needed forks
4. Count out needed knives
5. Count out needed napkins
6. Count out needed glasses
7. Place 1 plate in front of each chair
8. Fold the napkins in half
9. Place 1 napkin on the left side of each plate
10. Place 1 fork on each napkin
11. Place 1 knife on the right side of each plate
12. Place 1 glass by each knife

Stringing Isolated Skills Together to Create a Sequence

Once your child has several isolated skills, you can start to string them together to make a sequence. For example, if your child knows how to get dressed in the morning and brush their teeth, your next step would be to create a morning routine. This would allow you to add some additional steps like putting their pajamas in the hamper, transitioning from their bedroom to the bathroom independently, and so on. Here is an example of a basic morning routine:

1. Take off pajamas
2. Put in hamper
3. Put on underwear
4. Put on shirt
5. Put on pants
6. Put on socks
7. Walk to bathroom
8. Brush teeth (you could write out the steps if your child is not doing them 100% independently, or leave just as "brush teeth")
9. Head downstairs to kitchen

Here is a more advanced version of that same routine:

1. Check time on clock
2. Finish breakfast by 7:30 A.M.
3. Go upstairs to bedroom
4. Get dressed
5. Brush teeth
6. Go back downstairs
7. Get backpack and lunch
8. Go to front door
9. Put on shoes
10. Put on jacket
11. Tell Mom you are ready for the bus

You can see in this sequence that there are more steps, as well as the additional skills of time management and notifying Mom. Also note that some of the more specific steps are not listed in this routine—for example, putting on specific clothing items or walking to the bathroom. At this level, the simpler skills have been previously mastered and do not need to be listed. This allows you to focus on building upon the previously taught skills.

A task analysis can be applied to many different skills and help you to pinpoint where your child is struggling within a sequence, why they are struggling, and how to help them. Yes, this is a lot of information! With time, practice, and patience, you and your child will both learn new things. We know we are asking a lot, but the short-term effort can lead to long-term gains and quality-of-life improvements. Your child may want to be independent as much as you want them to be. We know this can be overwhelming—both the amount of information in this chapter as well as the ability to implement it in real life. Take some time to process it, do some self-care, and then come back to it, because this chapter is your ticket to your child's independence— and to your own. There will be a lot of bumps in the beginning, but stay with it and over time you'll see progress.

8

"How Do I Get Myself Out of the Routine?"

FADING PROMPTS TO BUILD INDEPENDENCE

Sara looked at her son Tony's evening routine task analysis data sheet for the week. The good news was that Tony had successfully completed his evening routine every day this week. The not-so-good news was that he would only do the routine when Sara was in sight. Sara knew Tony had made huge strides and was doing more of the routine independently than when they had first implemented the task analysis, but now she wanted to fade herself from the routine even more. The goal was for Tony to eventually be able to go upstairs and complete the routine on his own while Sara finished cleaning up after dinner. Sara wasn't sure how to get from where they were currently to where they wanted to be.

Now that you've learned about types of prompting (Chapter 6) and how to make a task analysis (Chapter 7), we're going to have you combine these skills. Once you and your child are successfully using one task analysis with one routine for at least a few weeks, we can start to think about how you can reduce the number and types of prompts you provide throughout your child's routine. The goal of this chapter is to reduce the number or level of prompts to move your child closer to independence and begin to fade yourself slowly out of the routine.

Fading is just like it sounds: It's reducing your role slowly over time. Think about receding into the background of the routine instead of being at

Fading Prompts to Build Independence

the forefront. Fading takes time, needs to be systematic, and requires accurate data so you know when to lower your level of support. Reducing the number of prompts and the intrusiveness of prompts allows your child more independence and decreases your involvement in their routines. This also helps you avoid the problem of prompt dependency.

As we've stated before, once a young adult exits the education system, many supports disappear unless they are paid for privately. Even then, finding support providers can be difficult, particularly for self-care tasks. Teaching these independent skills early and then slowly removing yourself from the routine helps your child build independence at a younger age. Starting early also gives your child more opportunities to practice the skill, and gives you opportunities to teach your child appropriate boundaries around these routines. We don't often have other adults in the bathroom with us when we brush our teeth, so your child shouldn't have people there either unless they're needed. We're hopeful that your child won't need other people around to complete these tasks after you fade yourself from the routine.

To get started, you'll first need an accurate count of the number of prompts you're providing and the types of prompts you're giving your child. This is your starting place, or baseline. For this, you'll bring back the task analysis for the routine you choose to work on first from Chapter 7, and use it for the "Getting the Full Prompting Picture" activity. Pull that task analysis out for your reference.

ACTIVITY: Getting the Full Prompting Picture

First, estimate how many of each type of prompt you will use during the routine so that your child can successfully complete it. Place those numbers in the table below. Remember that most people underestimate the amount of

	Less intrusive			More intrusive		
Type	Positional (P)	Model (M)	Gestural (G)	Verbal (V)	Partial physical (PP)	Full physical (FP)
Number of prompts used						

support they provide to their child during these routines. Their assistance has become so habitual that it is often unconscious.

Now comes the doing part. Go ahead and complete this routine with your child while recording yourself and your child on your smart device. Then, go back to the video and make tallies in the boxes below for each type of prompt you give to your child. Let's see how close you were to your original estimate.

Type	Less intrusive			More intrusive		
	Positional (P)	Model (M)	Gestural (G)	Verbal (V)	Partial physical (PP)	Full physical (FP)
Number of prompts used						

How did it go? Did you use fewer or more prompts than you thought? How about the types of prompts? Did you use more from the less intrusive side or the more intrusive side? Was that what you expected?

Fading with Joshua and Aiden

Now on to the "how to" of the fading part. There are two ways you can go about reducing or fading prompts. You can reduce the number of prompts. For example, five partial physical prompts may be reduced down to two partial physical prompts. You can also move the prompts farther down the hierarchy or, in other words, reduce their intrusiveness. For example, six full physical prompts may be decreased down to two partial physical prompts and four gestural prompts.

Just like in some other chapters, we will go through a series of vignettes to illustrate the fading process for you. Let's look at the mealtime routine for Joshua and his son Aiden. Joshua is going to give this his best shot, but he doesn't yet know what you now know from reading this book. Read this first vignette with your most critical eye. Bring all the knowledge you have acquired through reading this book about how to set your child up for success. Try to find all the places that Joshua either missed an opportunity to teach his son, or even did something that will likely lead to increased prompt dependence. Also look for the successes. What things did Joshua do right? What strategies and prompts do you recognize from earlier in the book?

Joshua really wants his 10-year-old son with autism, Aiden, to take a bigger role in family routines. Joshua's other children started doing chores around the house at a young age. They also started making themselves small snacks and helping clean up after dinner. This all came together after talking to Aiden's speech therapist about natural social opportunities to practice pragmatic language. Joshua realized that Aiden was missing out on some important social time with family and quite a few independent living skills because he wasn't expected to help with mealtimes. Joshua and Aiden's mom, Amelia, have been focused on other things with Aiden, but Joshua knows that they need to increase their expectations. Usually, Aiden gets to play in his room until Joshua or Amelia calls him to dinner. He gets to eat as quickly as he wants and then he can leave the table. This isn't how mealtimes go at school, at restaurants, or in any other social meal situation. Joshua and Amelia figure they can add Aiden to the routine just like they did with their other kids. Joshua let his other two kids know that Aiden was going to start setting the table and making the salad on Tuesday and Thursday nights. Let's watch Joshua start working with Aiden on mealtime tasks.

The First Try

Joshua notes that it's about 15 minutes before dinner is ready. He calls up to Aiden's room, "Hey, bud, it's time to help with dinner." After 30 seconds, Aiden doesn't respond. Joshua trudges up the stairs and finds Aiden watching a YouTube video on his tablet. Joshua says again, "Aiden, you're going to help with dinner tonight. Come on." Aiden says, "Now?" Joshua replies, "Yeah, bud, right now." There is some initial whining, which Joshua ignores. Then he says, "Okay, let's go to the kitchen," and steers Aiden by the shoulders toward the stairs. Once in the kitchen, Joshua says, "First we're going to set the table." Aiden stands in the doorway. Joshua says, "Get out five forks and five spoons." Aiden continues to stand in the doorway. Joshua moves closer to Aiden and guides him to the drawer, nudges his arm toward the drawer, and says, "Pull it open." Aiden opens the drawer and grabs a handful of forks and spoons. Joshua stops him and says, "Put those back and count out five." Aiden puts the silverware back and counts out five forks and spoons on the countertop. Joshua persists. "Okay, now take the forks and spoons over to the table. Grab five napkins and put them down first." After watching Aiden struggle with that multistep direction, Joshua repeats himself. Joshua walks over and demonstrates how to put the napkin down and places a spoon and fork on top. Then he moves the napkin setup to line up with the chair. "See?" he says. "Just like this." Aiden lays down the napkin and then puts a fork and a spoon facing upside down. Joshua pulls the example setup back in front of Aiden and says, "Make it look like this." Aiden moves the utensils into the correct position after a few tries. "Nice work!" and a high five from Joshua follow. Now Joshua says, "Time to get out glasses. How many do we need?" Aiden replies, "I don't know." Joshua helps Aiden count how many table settings there are. When they reach five, Joshua says, "That's right, buddy!" Aiden goes to the cabinet and gets five glasses. Joshua says, "Now put a glass by each fork." When Aiden is finished, Joshua says, "Okay, time to make the salad . . ." He glances up. By this point, Amelia has called the other kids to supper and has the soup heated on the stove. Joshua decides that he'll just make the salad quickly. He says, "Aiden, go ahead and sit down. I'll make the salad."

Answer Key to the First Try

Joshua notes that it's about 15 minutes before dinner is ready. He calls up to Aiden's room, "Hey, bud, it's time to help with dinner" (*verbal prompt*). After 30 seconds, Aiden doesn't respond. Joshua trudges up the stairs and finds Aiden watching a YouTube video on his tablet. Joshua says again, "Aiden, you're going to help with dinner tonight. Come on" (*verbal prompt and proximity*). Aiden says, "Now?" Joshua replies, "Yeah, bud, right now." There is some initial whining, which Joshua ignores. Then he says, "Okay, let's go to the kitchen," and steers Aiden by the shoulders toward the stairs (*verbal and physical prompt at shoulders*). Once in the kitchen, Joshua says, "First we're going to set the table" (*verbal prompt—nonspecific direct prompt*). Aiden stands in the doorway. Joshua says, "Get out five forks and five spoons" (*verbal prompt—specific and direct*). Aiden continues to stand in the doorway. Joshua moves closer to Aiden and guides him to the drawer (*physical prompt at shoulder*), nudges his arm toward the drawer, and says, "Pull it open" (*verbal and physical prompt at elbow*). Aiden opens the drawer and grabs a handful of forks and spoons. Joshua stops him (*physical prompt at hands*) and says, "Put those back and count out five" (*verbal prompt*). Aiden puts the silverware back and counts out five forks and spoons on the countertop. Joshua persists. "Okay, now take the forks and spoons over to the table. Grab five napkins and put them down first" (*verbal prompt*).

After watching Aiden struggle with that multistep direction, Joshua repeats himself (*verbal prompt*). Joshua walks over and demonstrates how to put the napkin down and places a spoon and fork on top (*model prompt*). Then he moves the napkin setup to line up with the chair. "See?" he says. "Just like this" (*model and verbal prompt*). Aiden lays down the napkin and then puts a fork and a spoon facing upside down. Joshua pulls the example setup back in front of Aiden and says, "Make it look like this" (*model and verbal prompt*). Aiden moves the utensils into the correct position after a few tries. "Nice work!" and a high five from Joshua follow (*reinforcement*). Now Joshua says, "Time to get out glasses. How many should we need?" (*verbal prompt*). Aiden replies, "I don't know." Joshua helps Aiden count how many table settings there are (*verbal prompt*). When they reach five, Joshua says, "That's right, buddy!" (*reinforcement*). Aiden goes to the cabinet and gets five glasses. Joshua says, "Now put a glass by each fork" (*verbal prompt*). When Aiden is finished, Joshua says, "Okay, time to make the salad . . . " (*verbal prompt*). He glances up. By this point, Amelia has called the other kids to supper and has the soup heated on the stove. Joshua decides that he'll just make the salad quickly. He says, "Aiden, go ahead and sit down. I'll make the salad" (*verbal prompt*).

Okay, let's check back in. Did you find all the mistakes (and successes!) in the routine? Think about the strategies that Joshua probably already knew about but that get lost in the day-to-day routines: avoiding verbal prompts, making sure to follow through on directions, minimizing distractions, and giving one direction at a time.

Task Analysis and Prompting to the Rescue . . . ?

Joshua felt ready. With the help of *Spectrum of Independence: How to Teach Your Neurodiverse Child Daily Life Skills*, he had made a task analysis for his son Aiden to take part in the family mealtime routine (setting the table, making a simple salad, and putting the dishes in the sink afterward). He knew all the types of prompts he should and could provide to his son. He tried to remember to avoid verbal prompts and knew that the major struggle for Aiden was initiating the first step of the routine. Joshua and Amelia also discussed Aiden needing more practice opportunities, so they made setting the table and making the salad Aiden's chore each night. Joshua also knows that dinner is a powerful motivator for making sure setting the table and making a salad are taken care of quickly. Here's how it was going.

Before Aiden went up to his room, Joshua reminded him, "Hey, Aiden, you're setting the table tonight at 6, so that's in 30 minutes. You have 30 minutes to play on your tablet." Joshua called up to Aiden one time before then, warning him that he had 5 minutes left. Right at 6:00, Joshua walked into Aiden's room and told him to turn off the tablet. Then Joshua said, "Time to go downstairs to set the table and make the salad." Aiden had stopped whining about the chore sometime in the first three weeks, but wasn't exactly eager to get started. When they entered the kitchen, Joshua pointed at the written task analysis that sat on the table. He read out the first step. When Aiden didn't move, Joshua physically guided him to the area needed. After each step, Aiden stopped and looked at his dad for a prompt. Joshua read every step out loud and gave physical or modeling guidance for the task. They'd added all of the salad-making routine steps to the task analysis too. Joshua was sure that Aiden could do more, but he couldn't figure out how to get himself out of the routine. He'd heard the term prompt dependency and wondered if that was what had happened with Aiden.

Prompt Fading: Moving toward Independence

We provide descriptions of four ways to begin to fade yourself out of the routines you are working on with your child. Each method involves collecting data on the type of prompt you are using, deciding what fading procedure to use, and then implementing that procedure. You can also fade by implementing the prompt below that one in the hierarchy. For example, if you're using model prompts, you would lower the prompt level to gestural prompts. So, instead of showing your child how to open the drawer, pick up a fork, and pick up a knife, you can point at the silverware drawer, then point at the forks and knives.

Time Delay

Time delay involves exactly what it sounds like, delay for a certain amount of time. This means pausing before you provide a prompt. You can pause for between one and five seconds. If your child is motivated to finish the routine, then the delay will also motivate them to complete the step on their own rather than waiting for you. This isn't a failsafe, but it's a great place to start and relatively easy for you to do. Simply count in your head slowly to your delay time before providing the prompt that your child is used to receiving at each step. Once your child does not require any physical prompts, you can also work to increase your distance from your child while you give gestural, model, or positional prompts. Time delay can also be used in conjunction with any prompt. You can pause before providing a prompt to see if your child will initiate the action independently.

Written, Visual, and Video Prompts

When we think about the future for your child, the less intrusive the prompts, the better. As adults, we use written, visual, and video prompts in our everyday life. The grocery list we make, the "No Parking" sign we see near the fire hydrant, and the YouTube video we watch on how to fix some small issue around the house, can all be viewed as prompts. These are prompts that your child can carry forward with them into whatever living situation suits them best.

Written prompts can be used for children who can read, while visual and video prompts can be used for children who cannot read yet or in situations when you want to lower the cognitive load of a task for children who can read. Visuals can include pictures of the actual objects in use during the routine, drawings of those objects, or representations of the action taking place in each step. For example, for the salad-making routine that Aiden uses, the first step could be a picture of the refrigerator. The second picture could be of the refrigerator with the door open and the vegetable drawer open. The third picture could be of the salad spinner. The fourth picture could be of Aiden (or a sibling) pulling the greens out of a container to put into the salad spinner. For a written version, you would write out the specific steps (open refrigerator, open vegetable drawer, take out salad container, put salad container on the counter, get out salad spinner from the cabinet, put salad spinner on the counter, open salad container, put the salad into the salad spinner, turn on cold-water tap, run salad spinner under water, turn off tap, pour out water, put lid on salad spinner, spin salad).

For a video model, you would record someone your child knows (you, the child's other parent, a sibling) completing the routine. Think of the video as one long model prompt. Your child can watch it as many times as they need, rewinding and rewatching. In research, video models have been helpful for adaptive skills, social skills, and play skills for people with disabilities ages 5–22 years old (Wong et al., 2015).

Electronic Prompts

One way to fade yourself out of routines is to provide prompts using technology. Let's think about the morning routine. If the end goal is for your child to get up in the morning independently, you could add wake-up calls from electronic assistants like Siri and Alexa, apps that start a slow wake-up routine, or child-friendly alarm clocks. Your child likely has scheduling demands and transitions throughout the day that you are managing for them. This will eventually need to transition from parent-led to child-led. This is the difference between you saying, "It's time for karate" and your child knowing it is time for karate without you reminding them. Apps and electronic assistants can be programmed to give announcements at different times throughout the day to prompt different routines. For example, Alexa can announce the end of TV time and the start of the dinner routine. It's important to remember that you will need to be ready to follow through on the prompt provided by the electronic assistant until your child learns to respond to the electronic prompt.

If your child can't tell time, timers are a great way to make time visual and auditory. There are products like visual timers that allow your child to see the passage of time. You can also teach your child to set timers and reminders for themselves. For example, if you tell them they have 15 minutes to play before it's time to leave for the park, they can set their own 15-minute timer verbally ("Alexa, set a 15-minute timer") or they can use a smartwatch or timer manually.

Setting up the Environment for Independence

There are quite a few ways to set up an environment to support independence. We give some ideas for each routine that you've heard before in previous chapters. First, you can ensure that all needed materials are visible at the start of the routine or are clearly labeled for your child. For example, put the toothbrush out on the counter, on a stand, or in the cup your child uses to rinse out their mouth. Many adults use these as prompts too! For the nighttime routine, make sure your child's drawers are labeled with pictures or written text to show where pj's and underwear are located. During the after-school routine, label the spot for your child to put their backpack and their shoes when they come in from school. These examples demonstrate how we use cues in the environment to transfer your child's reliance on you for the next step of a routine to the environment for that information instead. Eventually, the labels may be faded out. You can do this by making the labels smaller and smaller over time or removing certain labels as your child masters the skills within a given routine.

Prompt Dependency

Prompt dependency is a phenomenon where someone becomes dependent on a prompt, rather than completing an activity by themselves. This can happen to anyone. Think about the kid who waits until their parent asks about homework before even looking in their backpack or the husband who has to be told each week to take out the trash. What about the roommate who needs someone to ask for their half of the rent before they pay it or the coworker who needs constant reminders to get things in on time? These people are prompt dependent for at least this one part of their lives. For those people, there are natural consequences for not following through on their obligations. They might get a zero on their homework, have to deal with the smell of two-week-old trash or an overflowing trash bin, get charged a late fee by their landlord, or be put on an action plan at work. However, those consequences may come too late to influence their behavior in the moment.

Now think back to our section on reinforcement from Chapter 5. For a child with a disability, many consequences may be too far removed for them to connect to their lack of action. You and I can see how not brushing our teeth can lead to cavities, but still rely on the receptionist at the dentist office to prompt us to make a follow-up appointment. Prompt dependency could also come from the brief break a child gets between steps of a routine or before starting a routine. That's why we start with the least intrusive prompt they need to be successful, so we don't create prompt dependency. This also means decreasing or fading your prompts as quickly as you can. If your child has been successful with a prompt for three days, that is a good time to decrease to a lower type of prompt. Now let's check back in with Joshua and Aiden.

Fading Out

Thirty minutes before dinnertime, a preset announcement from an electronic assistant says, "Aiden, in five minutes, it will be time to go downstairs." Five minutes later, it dings and says, "Aiden, it's time to go set the table." Joshua waits at the bottom of the stairs and counts to 10. He started by standing at Aiden's bedroom door, then at the top of the stairs, and then to his new spot. He's hoping to fade himself so that he doesn't have to leave the kitchen to come get Aiden. Aiden tromps down the stairs as Joshua reaches 10. Joshua hands Aiden the task analysis as they walk to the kitchen together. The first time they went over the task analysis together, Joshua prompted Aiden to read each step, which he slowly faded out using time delay as Aidan showed more independence. Joshua would pause and count to three before providing the next prompt. Joshua says, "There are four of us having dinner tonight. Your sister has softball practice." Joshua points to the 4 written in dry-erase marker at the top of the laminated task analysis. Aiden asks, "Four forks and spoons?" Joshua points at the 4 again. Aiden looks at the task analysis and says, "Four napkins, four forks, four spoons, and four glasses." Aiden continues to follow the list, setting out the napkins, forks, spoons, and glasses. The only prompts that Joshua provides are gestural. If Aiden pauses for more than 10 seconds between tasks, Joshua points to the next step on the task analysis for Aiden to read out loud. When he is finished, Amelia says, "Aiden, that looks great! Thank you for setting the table for dinner!" Next on the list is prepping salad. Joshua has Aiden read each of the steps one at a time, and Joshua provides only model and gestural prompts. Amelia provides strong praise (a preferred reinforcer for Aiden!) once Aiden finishes the salad. Amelia also praises Aiden for doing the tasks more independently.

ACTIVITY: Targeting Prompts to Fade

Let's get into the details of pinpointing which prompts to fade first. Look back at your task analysis and see which steps require any type of physical prompt. These are the steps to fade first. You'll want to complete the routine at least once successfully before moving down the prompt list. If you're using a full physical prompt, try to fade back to a partial physical prompt. The fading process relies heavily on the use of a time delay. When you give your child a few extra seconds to respond, you can get a better feel for what they are able to do independently. This allows you to gauge what level of prompt they need. For example, you'll wait three seconds to see what (if anything) they attempt to do. If they do not initiate the next step, then use the least intrusive prompt necessary to complete the step.

Now that you have guidance on how to fade the prompts with examples from this chapter and Chapter 6, you can start to remove yourself slowly from one routine. Once you are completely removed, or removed to a level that makes sense for your child's age (most 8-year-olds still need to be reminded to brush their teeth, but most 15-year-olds should not), you can start working on your next routine. Before you begin to work on the second routine, take a moment to think about the progress you and your child have made so far. Think about (and even add up) the time you're saving. Consider any new things your child can do that they couldn't do before you started actively working with them to increase their independence. Allow yourself to contemplate the new horizons that this independence has opened for your child. Savor that progress and your success. The road to independence is long, and stopping to admire the view along the way can help you appreciate how far you've come!

Part V

Maximizing Independence

9

"When Do I Modify the Goal?"
ACCOMMODATING THE CHILD VERSUS MODIFYING THE GOAL

Lisa had gone out of her way to babyproof the house when Joey started to crawl. As he entered toddlerhood and became slightly more rambunctious, she rearranged the house again, moving things farther out of reach. As time went on, Lisa had installed locking cabinets, placed toddler-proof baby gates at the stairs, and moved all breakable items out of Joey's reach. She had also decreased clutter off the countertops in the bathrooms by putting away many items Joey needed.

Now that Joey was six, though, she wanted him to start doing more things for himself. She realized she'd have to un-babyproof some things. She had the toothpaste in the medicine cabinet where he could not reach it, and the soap in a pump soap container that he could not pump independently. His coat was supposed to be put on a hanger, which Joey could not do, and hung on a bar in the closet that Joey could not reach. Lisa also had all the snacks up high so that he needed to request them—but that was for when they were teaching him to request. Now that he knew how to request, she really wanted him to be able to get his own snack.

Lisa took some time the next morning while Joey was at school to make a few changes. She moved the toothpaste to the vanity so Joey could reach it. She put out a soap dispenser that was activated by a motion-based sensor. All Joey had to do was put his hand under it and it would squeeze out a small amount of soap. She hung a coat hook at Joey's level in the closet, and moved his snacks to a lower cabinet that he could access independently. All these changes would allow Joey to be more independent.

In our day jobs working with children with a developmental or intellectual disability, our goal is for them to be as independent *as possible.* That "as possible" part is pretty important. We want you to remember that this will look different for different children. For some children, this may mean being able to complete the entire task independently. Others may require the task itself to be modified in order for them to find success in completing it. Other children may be able to complete the original task if adaptations are made in *how* they complete the task. As with anything, there are drawbacks and positives to both ways of supporting your child. Some children require modification of the goal, while others require an accommodation in how they complete the goal. You may be asking yourself how to know which is appropriate for your child. Don't worry! It will all make sense with the strategies you'll learn in this chapter.

Now to define *modifications* and *accommodations.* The first goal of this chapter is for you to be clear about the difference between modifying a goal and accommodating your child. We want you to be aware of when you are using either technique, and understand when each should be used. The second goal of this chapter is learning to be cognizant of the consequences of modifications and accommodations. Although modifying a goal may make things easier in the moment, there are often undesirable consequences in the long run. You'll be able to gauge which is best for your child and their goals for lifelong independence.

Modifications

DEFINITION: A *modification* is when you change the end goal—in many cases, to make it easier. It is important to note that modifying a goal without a plan to teach the skills a child needs to eventually do the task on their own means accepting this level of functioning for the rest of that person's life.

EXAMPLES: Your child has a goal to take a shower independently, including washing their hair. They have motor delays that make it challenging for them to access the shampoo and conditioner. Additionally, they have trouble washing parts of their body that they can't reach. You modify the end goal so that they do not need to wash their hair and you accept that they will only wash part of their body with soap. This means that some other person will need to wash their hair and parts of their body for the foreseeable future.

WHEN TO USE: In the realm of this book and the population we are addressing, there would be very few, if any, times when modifying a daily living goal would be appropriate. However, in the grander scheme of life, there are times when modifications are appropriate. If your child has physical limitations, you may need to modify or assist with certain tasks. For example, many people with motor planning deficits and muscle weakness often struggle to complete fine motor activities like cutting their fingernails. Academically, if you have a child with an intellectual disability, there may be times when modifying classwork is appropriate. If you or your child are very ill with mono, the flu, or a stomach bug, or have some time-limited decrease in energy, you can also temporarily modify routines. We don't do the same things when we're sick as when we're healthy, and you can adjust accordingly.

The Difference between Modifications and Prompts

You may be asking, what is the difference between a modification and a prompt? If you are, that is a great question! For starters, you modify a goal, but you prompt a person. When you modify a goal, you change the goal, usually by making it easier. For example, instead of having your child brush all of their teeth for two minutes, you accept that they are only brushing the front four teeth for five seconds. This lowers the performance requirements needed by your child to meet the goal. You can change a modification to make it "less modified," for example, setting a timer and insisting they keep the toothbrush in their mouth for two minutes even though they are still only brushing the front four teeth. However, you can't fade a modification the way you fade a prompt, because you have not taught your child how to improve the skill. Compare this to when you prompt your child. When you prompt your child, you are helping them to reach the original goal—for example, showing them with hand-over-hand prompts how to brush each quadrant of their mouth so that all of their teeth get cleaned. And, as an added bonus, if you follow the prompt-fading techniques discussed in Chapter 8, then over time, you are also helping them learn how to complete the task independently.

In some cases, you may do a task for your child instead of

prompting them—for example, just brushing their teeth for them instead of showing them how to do it themselves. If your child is past the age or developmental level where they need you to do a task for them and you are still doing it for them, we consider this a modification as well. In this case, you have lowered your expectations of your child and removed the need for them to learn the skill.

There are many reasons why we may modify a goal or do a task for our child. Sometimes it's to make things easier for the child, sometimes it's to make things easier for you. There are cases when modifying is necessary, and then there are cases when it is done more out of convenience in that moment. The trick is to know the difference. This chapter will help you understand the nuances of both accommodating and modifying, and when to use each.

Accommodations

DEFINITION: An *accommodation* is when you make a daily living goal attainable by providing adaptations in how the goal can be completed. There are various ways to provide an accommodation. You can alter how the task is presented (presentation), how the child responds (response), the setting in which the task is presented (setting), and the time in which the child must complete the task (scheduling and time management). See the table on page 183.

EXAMPLES: A child has a goal to take a shower independently, including washing their hair. They have motor delays that make it challenging for them to access the shampoo and conditioner. Additionally, they have trouble washing parts of their body that they can't reach. You accommodate them by buying shampoo and conditioner dispensers that are activated by a motion sensor, and a loofah with a long handle for them to reach their back. You teach them to use the dispensers and the loofah so they can be independent in showering.

WHEN TO USE: Accommodations should be used whenever your child is struggling to complete a task or routine independently despite efforts to teach them to do so. For example, there is no need to accommodate your child

Type of accommodation	Daily living examples	Academic examples
Presentation	Creating a visual schedule for your child to help keep them on track during a daily living routine	Reading the directions of a math test to a child who has trouble reading
Response	Utilizing adaptive equipment like shampoo pumps, toothpaste dispensers, and large-handled knives	Allowing a child to respond to test questions orally instead of in writing
Setting	Organizing your child's clothes in a manner that they can reach everything they need and only have access to weather-appropriate clothes	Having a child sit close to the board
Scheduling and time management	Teaching your child to set timers if they do not know how to tell time so they can be responsible for their time management	Allowing a child to have extra time to complete a test

with a toothpaste dispenser if you have never attempted to teach them how to squeeze the appropriate amount of toothpaste out of the container. However, if after many attempts to teach these skills your child is still unsuccessful, it may be time to accommodate them. Remember, the ultimate goal is to fade yourself out of their daily living routines. If buying a toothpaste dispenser allows your child to complete the task on their own after failed attempts to teach them to use a regular toothpaste tube, then it is an appropriate accommodation.

More Examples of Modifications and Accommodations

There are many ways to provide accommodations and modifications. Here is just a small sample of some examples. Again, notice how the modifications alter the daily living goal so that the goal itself has been changed and the higher-level goal can no longer be met. Notice how the accommodations factor in the child's ability level; changes are made to presentation, setting, response, or schedule, but the goal remains unchanged.

Behavior

Modifications	Accommodations
Allowing your child to not clean their room or having someone do it for them	Setting up your child's room (e.g., labeled drawer system, removing nonessential items) so that they can be responsible for keeping it clean
Not exposing your child to new foods because of the tantrum or pushback that it will likely cause	Working with your child to discover new foods they may like and how different preparation methods may affect the outcome
Allowing your child to run around at sports practice aimlessly because they are having trouble following the group	Temporarily providing your child with an aide to help them learn the routine of practice so they can stay with the group
Allowing your neurodiverse child more time on electronics than you allow your neurotypical children because he doesn't enjoy any other activities	Ensuring that you have developmentally appropriate activities available, take the time to teach them to your child, and set rules for how much time can be spent on electronic versus nonelectronic activities
Allowing your child to request items by yelling	Accepting that your child may have limited speech, but insisting that they use a calm voice when requesting
Physically turning the TV off to let your child know that they need to stop watching TV	Setting a timer and teaching your child to be responsible for turning off the TV

Motor

Modifications	Accommodations
Hanging up your child's jacket for them because they cannot get their jacket on the hanger	Installing a hook in the closet for your child to put away their jacket independently

Accommodating the Child versus Modifying the Goal

Modifications	Accommodations
Allowing your child to dump half a bottle of shampoo onto the shower floor every night because they don't know how to squeeze the appropriate amount into their hand	Buying a pump shampoo bottle and teaching them that they only need one pump of shampoo
Putting your child's pants on for them because they have a hard time doing it themselves	Working with a physical therapist to figure out ways to make it easier for your child to put on their own pants, for example, having them sit on a stool instead of standing or sitting on the floor
Cutting your child's food for them	Buying an adaptive knife and teaching your child how to cut their own food
Zipping your child's jacket for them because they can't maneuver the small zipper	Buying your child a jacket that has fasteners that your child can maneuver independently—like a larger zipper, hooks, or snaps

Sensory

Modifications	Accommodations
Letting your child wear whatever they want to a fancy event	Buying your child a tagless collared shirt, made out of soft material, so he can be dressed appropriately for the event
Letting your child refuse to keep themselves clean	Allowing your child the choice of taking a bath or a shower
Not attending birthday parties because your child does not like the clapping after they sing "Happy Birthday"	Taking your child to a party but stepping out when the kids sing "Happy Birthday"
Letting your child run around at a party because he is overstimulated by the noise	Respecting that your child becomes overstimulated at loud events, proactively teaching them calming techniques, and accepting that they may not be able to attend the entire party, or will need breaks in a quiet room throughout the party to regroup

Modifications	Accommodations
Allowing your child to eat a limited diet because he has sensory issues with food	Working with a feeding or behavior specialist to create a plan that introduces new foods in a productive and systematic manner
Waking up your child every morning because they do not like the sound of the alarm clock	Buying an alarm clock that uses music or light instead of a buzzer

Academic

Modifications	Accommodations
Giving an easier test (e.g., fewer answer choices, fewer questions, covering less material than everyone else)	Giving the same test, but allowing extra time
Accepting that your child is not given homework because they are in a special education class, even though all the other students in the school receive homework	Requesting developmentally appropriate homework be sent home so they can learn how to be responsible for completing homework
Giving a child with a visual impairment a lower-level book to read because it has less words and larger font	Ordering the same book the rest of the class is reading in larger font or as audio
Giving more specific directions than what is printed in the test	Reading the same directions that are on the test
Assigning an easier, more condensed version of a large multistep project	Assigning the same large multistep project and scheduling weekly meetings to check in on the student's progress

Keeping Your Eye on the Prize

Why the Ultimate Goal Is Accommodation

In order to maximize your child's ability to live an independent life, we want to focus on making accommodations over modifications. Why? Well, out in the world, there are many situations that can be accommodated, but modification may not be possible. And what do we mean by "the real world"? Situations like general education classes, inclusive higher education programs, competitive employment, and independent living arrangements are a few examples.

Let's look at some real-world examples that you as an adult may come across.

- Completing an intake form at a doctor's office: Someone could help you write in the answers if you know all the answers, but the likelihood that the office would give you a modified form that requests less information is pretty unlikely.

- Completing a task at work: If you are employed at a nonsheltered (competitive and integrated) job, it is likely that you will need to complete your tasks at the same level of proficiency as your neurotypical coworkers. Although your boss may accommodate you by being flexible in how you complete your work, it is likely that the finished product will need to reach a common level of quality and be completed on a similar timeline as your coworkers.

- Getting dressed to go to work: Although dress codes in work environments have significantly dwindled, there are still many professions that require employees to show up dressed in business attire (collared shirt and tie, blouse and dress pants) or a specific uniform (barista at a coffee shop, waiter at a restaurant, equipment checkout worker at a chain gym, salesperson at a store). Although a person may be accommodated with the allowance of softer fabric, tagless clothes, and so on, the likelihood that the boss will allow one person to ignore the dress code is pretty slim.

As you can see, it is much easier to function in the world if you do not need to rely on modifications.

Now let's look at some real-world examples you may come across with your child.

- You want your child to independently pack a healthy lunch for school. Most mornings you pack it for them, because if you let them pack it, all they want to bring is junk food. You could continue to pack it for them (modification) or accept that they are bringing unhealthy foods to school (modification). You could also take a different approach and stock up on healthy snacks, remove the junk food, and explain that they need to choose one item from each of three different groups of food (one fruit, one healthy snack, one drink). This would be considered an accommodation.

- You want your child to put their shoes on independently. You bought them high-tops that are really hard to get on, so you have to do it for them. You could continue to do it for them (modification), or you could buy them regular sneakers that they are able to put on themselves (accommodation). If you choose to buy them regular sneakers, you could continue to teach them how to put on their high-tops outside of the morning routine using a shoehorn (accommodation).

- You want your child to eat a healthy breakfast, but they will only eat one specific sugary cereal. You could allow them to eat the cereal (modification), or you could create a plan to systematically introduce healthier breakfast foods (accommodation) and fade out the sugary cereal.

By starting to incorporate the use of accommodations early on instead of relying on modifications, you set your child up for success both now and later on in life.

Vignette 1

This first vignette follows mom Sara and her 10-year-old son Thomas as they move through his evening routine. This vignette illustrates the routine before Sara has learned about accommodations and modifications. Read through and see if you can identify the accommodations and modifications that Sara uses. As a bonus, see if you can also identify the prompts Sara uses!

> It is 7:00 P.M. Sara calls to her 10-year-old son Thomas in the living room, "Put away your toys, it's time to take a shower." Thomas, either unaware of her yells or not wanting to stop playing, continues to play. Five minutes later, Sara walks into the living room and starts putting his toys away in the bins while narrating, "Cars go with cars, and blocks go with blocks. Time to clean up." Thomas throws himself on the floor and starts to whine, "No! I want to play more! I just started playing." Sara ignores his complaints and repeats that it is time to take a shower as she points to the stairs. Thomas lets out one more groan, gets up off the floor, and stomps his way up the stairs

and into the bathroom. Sara walks into the bathroom a few moments later and sees Thomas playing with some minifigures on the counter instead of brushing his teeth. Sara ups the pep in her voice and says, "Put those down and brush your teeth." Thomas puts toothpaste on the toothbrush and puts the toothbrush in his mouth. He starts to move it around a bit, but then says, "Finished!" after only a few seconds. Sara doesn't have it in her to argue with him about it tonight, so she lets it go. Then she says, "Shower time," and points toward the bathtub. He stands by the sink and tries to unbutton his pants unsuccessfully. Sara hopes he will eventually ask for help, but he just starts getting frustrated. To avoid another whining spell, she unbuttons the button on his pants for him. Then she turns on the shower. Once she regulates the temperature, Thomas gets into the shower and gets himself wet. In the past, Sara had tried to teach him how to wash his body, but between spilling the liquid soap everywhere, only washing parts of his body, and getting distracted throughout, it always ended up with her having to rewash him anyway. Due to her exhaustion by that time at night, and in the interest of time, most nights it is easier for Sara to wash him herself than trying to show him how to do it. She is slightly concerned about this, as Thomas is about to turn 11 and is finally starting to want more privacy, which is a relief, since he has already started puberty. Sara is not sure how to fade herself from the shower routine without allowing him to do an inadequate job of washing himself, not to mention she doesn't want him to experience the social consequences of being "the smelly kid" at school. As she washes him, Sara thinks about all the things she'd tried previously to help Thomas be more independent and to make taking a shower easier. She'd tried to teach him how to put the shampoo in his hand, but he always ended up getting way more than he needed. She had also tried to get him a pump bottle for the shampoo, but there wasn't a shelf to put it on, Thomas had a hard time getting the bottle from the shower caddy, and she still needed to help him regardless. After she puts the shampoo in his hand, he is able to lather up his short hair, but he isn't great about actually scrubbing his scalp, particularly near his ears and the back of his neck. She double-checks to make sure he actually got shampoo on those areas. Nope, no shampoo suds there. Once she scrubs those areas, she rinses him off and turns off the water. Thomas can mostly dry himself independently, but sometimes she helps him just to speed things up because she knows she has a good 30-minute battle ahead of her to get him dressed and into bed. Once he is dry, he takes off down the hall naked to his bedroom. He is supposed to put on his pajamas, which she had already laid out on his bed. Instead, he is looking at a book on his bed. She takes the book away and points to his pajamas. He has trouble putting them on because they are tight, but he also isn't in a rush to get dressed because what comes next is bedtime—and he doesn't particularly enjoy going to bed. In fact, Sara finds that he becomes really silly at this point in the evening and has a hard time settling down, often leading to a stressful and late end to both of their days. Sara puts his pajamas on for him and then engages in their usual "game" of trying to wrestle him into bed.

Answer Key to Vignette 1

It is 7:00 P.M. Sara calls to her 10-year-old son Thomas in the living room, "Put away your toys, it's time to take a shower." Thomas, either unaware of her yells or not wanting to stop playing, continues to play. Five minutes later, Sara walks into the living room and starts putting his toys away in the bins (*modification*) while narrating, "Cars go with cars, and blocks go with blocks (*verbal prompt*). Time to clean up (*verbal prompt*)." Thomas throws himself on the floor and starts to whine, "No! I want to play more! I just started playing." Sara ignores his complaints and repeats that it is time to take a shower as she points to the stairs (*gestural prompt*). Thomas lets out one more groan, gets up off the floor, and stomps his way up the stairs and into the bathroom (*modification*). Sara walks into the bathroom a few moments later and sees Thomas playing with some minifigures on the counter instead of brushing his teeth. Sara ups the pep in her voice and says, "Put those down and brush your teeth (*verbal prompt*)." Thomas puts toothpaste on the toothbrush and puts the toothbrush in his mouth. He starts to move it around a bit, but then says, "Finished!" after only a few seconds. Sara doesn't have it in her to argue with him about it tonight, so she lets it go (*modification*). Then she says, "Shower time," and points toward the bathtub (*verbal and gestural prompt*). He stands by the sink and tries to unbutton his pants unsuccessfully. Sara is hoping he'll eventually ask for help, but he just starts getting frustrated. To avoid another whining spell, she unbuttons the button on his pants for him (*modification*). Then she turns on the shower (*modification*). Once she regulates the temperature (*modification*), Thomas gets into the shower and gets himself wet. In the past, Sara had tried to teach him how to wash his body, but between spilling the liquid soap everywhere, only washing parts of his body, and getting distracted throughout, it always ended up with her having to rewash him anyway (*modification*). Due to her exhaustion by that time at night, and in the interest of time, most nights it is easier for Sara to wash him herself than trying to show him how to do it. She is slightly concerned about this as Thomas is about to turn 11 and is finally starting to want more privacy, which is a relief, since he has already started puberty. Sara is not sure how to fade herself from the shower routine without allowing him to do an inadequate job of washing himself, not to mention she doesn't want him to experience the social consequences of being "the smelly kid" at school. As she washes him, Sara thinks about all the things she has tried previously to help Thomas be more independent and to make taking a shower easier. She'd tried to teach him how to put the shampoo in his hand, but he always ended up getting way more than he needed. She had also tried to get him a pump bottle for the shampoo (*accommodation*), but there wasn't a shelf to put it on, and Thomas had a hard time getting the bottle from the shower caddy, so she still needed to help him regardless. After she puts the shampoo in his hand (*modification*), he is able to lather up his short hair, but he isn't great about actually scrubbing his scalp, particularly near his ears and the back of his neck. She double-checks to make sure he actually got shampoo on those areas. Nope, no shampoo suds there. Once she scrubs those areas (*modification*), she rinses him off (*modification*) and turns off the water (*modification*). Thomas can mostly dry himself independently, but sometimes she helps him just to speed things up (*modification*) because she knows she has a good 30-minute battle ahead of her to get him dressed and into bed. Once he is dry, he takes off down the hall naked to his bedroom (*modification*). He is supposed to put on his pajamas, which she has already laid out on his bed (*modification*). Instead, he is looking at a book on his bed. She takes the book away and points to his pajamas (*gestural prompt*). He has trouble putting them on because they are tight, but he also isn't in a rush to get dressed because what comes next is bedtime—and he doesn't particularly enjoy going to bed. In fact, Sara finds that he becomes really silly at this point in the evening and has a hard time settling down, often leading to a stressful and late end to both of their days. Sara puts his pajamas on for him (*modification*) and then engages in their usual "game" of trying to wrestle him into bed (*modification*).

Vignette 2

This vignette will check in on Sara and Thomas a few weeks later, after Sara has learned about the difference between accommodating and modifying. See if you can identify the steps she took to accommodate Thomas in order to foster a higher level of independence, and a smoother, more enjoyable evening routine for both of them. Again, as an added bonus, see if you can also identify the prompts Sara used during the routine!

It is 6:30 p.m. Sara calls to her 10-year-old son Thomas in the living room, "Put away your toys, it's time to take a shower." Thomas begins to pick up his toys. Ever since Sara rearranged his evening routine and lined up some fun activities to take place after his shower, he has been much more willing to engage in the shower routine. Thomas finishes cleaning up his toys and then takes off up the stairs and into the bathroom. Sara walks into the bathroom a few moments later and sees Thomas brushing his teeth. She had bought him an electric toothbrush with a built-in timer. She explains to Thomas that he needs to brush his teeth until the toothbrush goes off. If he keeps the toothbrush in his mouth until it goes off, he earns a token that he can "cash in" after his shower. Thomas does not immediately start undressing after brushing his teeth, so Sara points to the shower. She has stopped giving him verbal prompts during shower time as she is working hard to fade herself out of the routine. Thomas takes off his pants. Sara has replaced his button pants with pants that have a snap that he can unfasten himself. In the meantime, she asked Thomas's occupational therapist to work with Thomas in session so he can learn how to unfasten the button. Thomas removes the rest of his clothes and then turns on the shower. Sara has put a piece of tape on the wall as a visual cue for Thomas to know where to turn the knob to for warm water. This allows him to regulate the temperature himself. Thomas gets into the shower and gets himself wet. Although they have experienced past failures in trying to teach Thomas how to wash his hair, Sara has thought up a few other ideas. She bought a shampoo dispenser that sticks to the wall. This frees Thomas up from having to maneuver the container and only requires him to place one hand under the device to catch the soap while using his other hand to push a button. This allows him to get shampoo himself, instead of relying on Sara to get it for him. Although he still isn't great about scrubbing near his ears and the back of his neck, Sara got into the habit of physically prompting him to reach those areas instead of doing it for him. This way she is giving him the opportunity to learn how do it himself. Thomas rinses himself off and turns off the water. Now that they are starting the routine earlier and Thomas is going through it more quickly, there is enough time to let him dry himself. Sara knows he can do this part himself, so she backs up toward the doorway to start to create space between them in preparation for eventually fading her presence. Once

Thomas is dry, he heads to the door. Sara points at the towel. He picks it up and wraps it around himself before taking off down the hall to his bedroom. He walks over to his dresser and picks out a pair of pajamas. Sara has reorganized his dresser so he can access the clothes he needs. She has also replaced his tight pajamas with looser-fitting ones that he can easily put on himself. She even let him pick out the new pajamas and was surprised that he had an opinion about which ones he wanted. Thomas knows that if he gets dressed quickly, he will earn another token. Prior to making changes in the routine, this part had always been a struggle. However, between the new pajamas and the addition of a reinforcer at the end of the routine, Thomas was now getting dressed in a matter of minutes, completely independently. Once he is dressed, he puts his towel in the hamper, collects his tokens, and goes over to his choice board. Tonight he wants to use his tokens to earn five minutes of playtime with Sara and a storybook. What had previously been one of the most stressful parts of Sara's day has turned into the most enjoyable. And the best part was that Thomas seemed to really be enjoying his increased independence as well.

Answer Key to Vignette 2

It is 6:30 P.M. Sara calls to her 10-year-old son Thomas in the living room, "Put away your toys, it's time to take a shower" (*accommodation—allow for extra time*). Thomas begins to pick up his toys. Ever since Sara rearranged his evening routine and lined up some fun activities to take place after his shower, he has been much more willing to engage in the shower routine (*accommodation—order of activities; appropriate use of reinforcers*). Thomas finishes cleaning up his toys and then takes off up the stairs and into the bathroom. Sara walks into the bathroom a few moments later and sees Thomas brushing his teeth. She had bought him an electric toothbrush with a built-in timer (*accommodation*). She explains to Thomas that he needs to brush his teeth until the toothbrush goes off. If he keeps the toothbrush in his mouth until it goes off, he earns a token that he can "cash in" after his shower (*appropriate use of reinforcers*). Thomas does not immediately start undressing after brushing his teeth, so Sara points to the shower (*gestural prompt*). She has stopped giving him verbal prompts during the routine as she is working hard to fade herself out of the routine. Thomas takes off his pants. Sara has replaced his button pants with pants that have a snap that he can unfasten himself (*accommodation*). In the meantime, she asked Thomas's occupational therapist to work with Thomas in session so he can learn how to unfasten the button. Thomas removes the rest of his clothes and then turns on the shower. Sara put a piece of tape on the wall as a visual for Thomas to know where to turn the knob to for warm water (*accommodation*). This allows him to regulate the temperature himself. Thomas gets into the shower and gets himself wet. Although they have experienced past failures in trying to teach Thomas how to wash his hair, Sara has thought up a few other ideas. She bought a shampoo dispenser that sticks to the wall (accommodation). This frees Thomas up from having to maneuver the container and only requires him to place one hand under the device and use his other hand to push a button. This allows him to get shampoo himself, instead of relying on Sara to get it for him. Although he still isn't great about scrubbing near his ears and the back of his neck, Sara got into the habit of physically prompting him to reach those areas instead of doing it for him (*physical prompt*). This way she is giving him the opportunity to learn how do it himself. Thomas rinses himself off and turns off the water. Now that they are starting the routine earlier and Thomas is going through it more quickly, there is enough time to let him dry himself. Sara knows he can do this part himself, so she backs up toward the doorway to start to create space between them in preparation for eventually fading her presence. Once Thomas is dry, he heads to the door. Sara points at the towel (*gestural prompt*). He picks it up and wraps it around himself before taking off down the hall to his bedroom. He walks over to his dresser and picks out a pair of pajamas. Sara has reorganized his dresser so he can access the clothes he needs (*accommodation*). She has also replaced his tight pajamas with looser-fitting ones that he can easily put on himself (*accommodation*). She even let him pick out the new pajamas and was surprised that he had an opinion about which ones he wanted. Thomas knows that if he gets dressed quickly, he will earn another token (*appropriate use of reinforcers*). Prior to making changes in the routine, this part had always been a struggle. However, between the new pajamas and the addition of a reinforcer at the end of the routine, Thomas is now getting dressed in a matter of minutes, completely independently. Once he is dressed, he puts his towel in the hamper, collects his tokens, and goes over to his choice board. This night he wanted to use his tokens to earn five minutes of playtime with Sara and a storybook. What had previously been one of the most stressful parts of Sara's day had turned into the most enjoyable. And the best part was that Thomas seemed to really be enjoying his increased independence as well.

ACTIVITY: Are You a Modifier or an Accommodator?

Review your child's morning and evening routines. Identify any steps that you are modifying or doing for them. Then identify any steps where you have provided an accommodation. Ask yourself the following questions:

- Are the accommodations you are using increasing your child's independence?
- Are there any modifications that can be replaced with accommodations?
- Are there any activities that you are doing for them that you could be prompting them to do for themselves?

Hopefully you found this to be an empowering chapter—for you and your child! It might take multiple attempts to figure out successful ways to accommodate your child. If you stick with it and maintain the mindset that the goal is to accommodate your child instead of modifying your goal, you will likely eventually find not only a solution, but also a higher level of independence for your child, and less stress for you.

Epilogue

"How Do I Keep Moving Forward?"
EXPANDING YOUR CHILD'S INDEPENDENCE

Congratulations! You've made it to the end of the book! No small task for anyone these days, especially a parent with the immense responsibility of raising a neurodiverse child. We hope you feel that the time you have spent reading this book and working through the activities has been time well spent. We hope that the skills you have learned have been (and will continue to be) beneficial to both you and your child. And most of all, we hope that both you and your child get to experience the joys of your child's increased independence.

You may be wondering, "Now that I finished the book, what's next?" The skills you have learned throughout this book can be applied to many different daily living routines, and our hope is that you will continue to apply this knowledge to increase your child's independence through their day. We recommend repeating the activities and processes from Chapters 7–9 for any routine that your child uses daily (create a task analysis, determine the prompt level needed for success, fade prompts as your child becomes more independent). Then repeat for activities completed less often like performing weekly chores, getting ready for an after-school activity, or preparing for a family outing.

Think back to the beginning of this book and all the scary statistics about social skills, independent living, and employment. You've come a long way since then, and so has your child. Your willingness to think critically about your and your child's readiness, learn new concepts and apply them to your daily interactions with your child, and implement these evidence-based practices are a testament to your devotion to your child's success. We hope you are proud of yourself and how much progress you've made toward your long-term goal of independence for your child!

Glossary

Accommodation: Changes how a skill is taught or completed in order to make it more achievable; the skill itself is not altered, only how it is achieved

Applied behavior analysis (ABA): The application of the principles of learning theory to teach socially significant behavior

Autism spectrum disorder (ASD): A developmental disability characterized by challenges with social communication and repetitive or restrictive behaviors or interests

Backward chaining: A procedure that teaches the last step of a routine first, and then adds previous steps in the reverse order until the student can complete the entire routine

Behavioral momentum: When easier tasks are presented prior to the presentation of a more difficult task in order to build up momentum

Behavior analyst: Either a board certified behavior analyst (BCBA) or a licensed behavior analyst (LBA)

Board certified behavior analyst (BCBA): Professionals who are certified by the national Behavior Analysts Certification Board; BCBAs have at least a master's degree, have completed supervision hours, and have passed an exam prior to practicing behavior analysis

Chaining: A teaching procedure where complex routines are broken down into smaller steps that are linked together

Closed-ended activity: An activity that has a clear end (e.g., a puzzle, a board game, coloring a picture in a coloring book)

Consequence: The effect that follows a behavior (e.g., you scoop ice cream into a bowl (behavior) → you get to eat the ice cream (consequence); your child asks for a snack (behavior) → you get them a snack (consequence)

Contrived reinforcement: Reinforcement that is selected by a teacher or parent (e.g.,

Joey answers a question correctly, so the teacher gives him a star sticker); does not naturally occur following the child's behavior but is instead arranged ahead of time

Elopement: When a child leaves safe areas or safe people for any reason

Forward chaining: A procedure where the person is prompted to complete the first step and, upon mastery, subsequent steps are added

Individuals with Disabilities Education Act (IDEA): A law in the United States that states that all children, even those with disabilities, are entitled to a free and appropriate education

Intellectual disability (ID): A condition that affects brain development and a person's ability to function; generally determined with an IQ score under 70 and significantly lower adaptive skills

Intellectual or developmental disability (IDD): A condition that affects a person's intellectual functioning, in addition to their adaptive skills

Licensed behavior analyst (LBA): A behavior analyst that is licensed to practice applied behavior analysis in a specific state or states

Modification: Changes the skill that is taught by making the task easier; this changes the end goal and lowers the standard for the task

Natural reinforcement: Reinforcement that is connected to the behavior (e.g., receiving a cookie because you asked for a cookie; having another child laugh because you told a joke)

Negative reinforcement: A consequence that increases the future likelihood of a behavior by decreasing, removing, or delaying a stimulus (e.g., hitting your snooze button delays waking up and increases the likelihood you will hit snooze again; taking medicine removes your headache; giving your child what they want stops their crying)

Open-ended activity: An activity that does not have a clear ending (e.g., drawing a picture, playing with action figures, playing at a playground)

Positive reinforcement: A consequence that increases the future likelihood of a behavior by adding or increasing a stimulus (e.g., you ask for the music to be turned on and the driver of the car turns it up; you go to work and receive a paycheck)

Prerequisite skills: Skills that need to be mastered before another skill can be taught (e.g., learning letters before reading; learning how to speak before working on social conversation)

Probe: The initial presentation of a skill, without prompting, to see the learner's ability to engage in the skill

Prompt dependency: When a learner becomes so accustomed to being prompted that they not only expect it, but will wait for it instead of trying to complete tasks on their own

Punishment: A consequence that follows a behavior and decreases the future likelihood of that behavior occurring (e.g., when a child hits a classmate to get a toy, the teacher takes the toy away; the child is less likely to hit their peer to get a toy in the future)

Redirection: When a parent or teacher directs a learner to a more appropriate behavior in order to facilitate them stopping a (usually problem or incorrect) behavior they are engaged in (e.g., when John went to get into the bath, his mother redirected him to the sink to brush his teeth)

Reinforcement: a consequence that follow a behavior of interest and increases the future likelihood of the behavior (e.g., when a child whines to get a snack at the store, his father gives him the snack; the child is more likely to whine to get a snack in the future)

Routine: A series of events that occur together on a consistent basis

Section 504 of the Rehabilitation Act of 1973: A federal law that forbids discrimination against people with disabilities by federal agencies, federal contractors, and programs receiving federal funds; it also approves grants for vocational rehabilitation services, supported employment, and independent living

Self-regulation: A person's ability to regulate their emotions

Sensory (automatically) mediated behavior: Behavior that is brought on by and reinforced by something within the person; this behavior does not happen for social reasons (e.g., a child spins in circles while they are by themselves; their reinforcement for the behavior is the feeling they get from spinning)

Socially mediated behavior: Behavior that is brought on by and reinforced by something in the environment and outside of the child; the motivating functions of socially mediated behaviors are attention, tangible items or activities, or escape (e.g., a child cries for their parent's attention; their reinforcement for the behavior is the attention or comfort they receive from their parent)

Stereotypic behavior: Behavior that is automatically reinforced just by engaging in the behavior; usually repetitive in nature; see also **Sensory (automatically) mediated behavior**

Task analysis: The process of breaking down a skill or sequence into smaller, measurable, teachable units

References

Chan, W., Smith, L. E., Hong, J., Greenberg, J. S., Lounds Taylor, J., & Mailick, M. R. (2018). Factors associated with sustained community employment among adults with autism and co-occurring intellectual disability. *Autism, 22*(7), 794–803.

Dudley, C., Nicholas, D. B., & Zwicker, J. (2015). What do we know about improving employment outcomes for individuals with autism spectrum disorder? *SPP Research Paper, 8*(32). https://papers.ssrn.com/sol3/papers.cfm?abstract_id=2658823

Fair Labor Standards Act of 1938, 29 U.S.C. Ch. 8 (1938, revised 2011). *https://dol.gov/sites/dolgov/files/WHD/legacy/files/FairLaborStandAct.pdf*

Forbes, G., Kent, R., Charman, T., Baird, G., Pickles, A., & Simonoff, E. (2023). How do autistic people fare in adult life and can we predict it from childhood? *Autism Research, 16*(2), 458–473.

Gerhardt, P. F., & Lainer, I. (2011). Addressing the needs of adolescents and adults with autism: A crisis on the horizon. *Journal of Contemporary Psychotherapy, 41*, 37–45.

Human Services Research Institute & National Association of State Directors of Developmental Disabilities Services. (2019). *In-person survey 2017–2018 final report*. National Core Indicators. https://legacy.nationalcoreindicators.org/upload/core-indicators/17-18_IPS_National_Report_PART_I_update_CA_entitlement.pdf

Lippold, T., & Burns, J. (2009). Social support and intellectual disabilities: A comparison between social networks of adults with intellectual disability and those with physical disability. *Journal of Intellectual Disability Research, 53*(5), 463–473.

Majdalany, L., Wilder, D. A., Smeltz, L., & Lipschultz, J. (2016). The effect of brief delays to reinforcement on the acquisition of tacts in children with autism. *Journal of Applied Behavior Analysis, 49*(2), 411–415.

Mason, D., Capp, S. J., Stewart, G. R., Kempton, M. J., Glaser, K., Howlin, P., & Happé, F. (2021). A meta-analysis of outcome studies of autistic adults:

Quantifying effect size, quality, and meta-regression. *Journal of Autism and Developmental Disorders, 51,* 3165–3179.

Mazurek, M. O. (2014). Loneliness, friendship, and well-being in adults with autism spectrum disorders. *Autism, 18*(3), 223–232.

McCausland, D., McCallion, P., Carroll, R., & McCarron, M. (2021). The nature and quality of friendship for older adults with an intellectual disability in Ireland. *Journal of Applied Research in Intellectual Disabilities, 34*(3), 763–776.

Qian, X., Papay, C., Chaxiong, P., & Johnson, D. R. (2018). Literature review of employment outcomes for adults with intellectual and developmental disability. *International Review of Research in Developmental Disabilities, 55,* 213–266.

Roux, A. M., Shattuck, P. T., Rast, J. E., Rava, J. A., & Anderson, K. (2015). *National autism indicators report: Transition into young adulthood.* Life Course Outcomes Research Program, A. J. Drexel Autism Institute, Drexel University.

Sanford, C., Newman, L., Wagner, M., Cameto, R., Knokey, A. M., & Shaver, D. (2011). *The post-high school outcomes of young adults with disabilities up to 6 years after high school: Key findings from the National Longitudinal Transition Study-2 (NLTS2)* (NCSER 2011–3004). National Center for Special Education Research.

Tobin, M. C., Drager, K. D., & Richardson, L. F. (2014). A systematic review of social participation for adults with autism spectrum disorders: Support, social functioning, and quality of life. *Research in Autism Spectrum Disorders, 8*(3), 214–229.

U.S. Equal Employment Opportunity Commission. (2024). *2023 annual performance report.* www.eeoc.gov/2023-annual-performance-report

van Asselt-Goverts, A. E., Embregts, P. J. C. M., Hendriks, A. H. C., Wegman, K. M., & Teunisse, J. P. (2015). Do social networks differ? Comparison of the social networks of people with intellectual disabilities, people with autism spectrum disorders and other people living in the community. *Journal of Autism and Developmental Disorders, 45,* 1191–1203.

van Heijst, B. F., & Geurts, H. M. (2015). Quality of life in autism across the lifespan: A meta-analysis. *Autism, 19*(2), 158–167.

Wong, C., Odom, S. L., Hume, K. A., Cox, A. W., Fettig, A., Kucharczyk, S., . . . Schultz, T. R. (2015). Evidence-based practices for children, youth, and young adults with autism spectrum disorder: A comprehensive review. *Journal of Autism and Developmental Disorders, 45,* 1951–1966.

Index

Note. Boldface is used for entries found in the Glossary.

Academic functioning, 186. *See also* School setting
Accommodation. *See also* Modifications
   definition of, **199**
   as a goal over modifications, 186–195
   overview, 179–180, 182–186
   services after graduation and, 14
   struggles with task analysis and, 153
Activities of daily living, sequences for, 159–162. *See also* Daily living routines; Task analysis
Adaptive skills, 12, 24
Aggressive behaviors, 41–42, 47–48. *See also* Behaviors; Unsafe behaviors
Applied behavior analysis (ABA), **199**
Assessing for Barriers worksheet, 71, 76, 78, 79
Assessment. *See also* Readiness assessment
   child behavior safety assessment, 47–48
   foundational learning skills assessment, 58–59
   overview, 3
Attention functions of a behavior, 86, 88–89, 90, 100. *See also* Function of behaviors
Autism spectrum disorder (ASD), 12, 15–16, **199**
Automatically mediated behavior. *See* Sensory (automatically) mediated behavior

B

Backward chaining, 148–152, **199**. *See also* Chaining
Barriers
   assessing for, 71, 79
   task analysis and, 137, 139–146
Behavior analyst. *See also* Board Certified Behavior Analyst (BCBA)
   definition of, **199**
   elopement and, 43
   pica (eating nonfood items) and, 44
   self-injurious behavior and, 40–41
Behavioral data, 28–30
Behavioral momentum, 76, **199**
Behavioral vocabulary, 3, 24
Behaviors. *See also* Challenging or problem behavior; Function of behaviors; Sensory (automatically) mediated behavior; Socially mediated behavior; Unsafe behaviors
   consequences of, 95–100
   function of behaviors and, 86–95
   task analysis and, 24
Beliefs that your child is capable
   assessing, 72, 73, 77
   readiness of parents, 64, 69–70, 79
Bias, 18

205

Board Certified Behavior Analyst (BCBA). *See also* Behavior analyst
  definition of, **199**
  overview, 2, 12–13
Boundaries, 66
Brainstorming solutions, 71, 73, 76, 77, 78, 81
Brainstorming Solutions worksheet, 71, 76, 77, 78, 81
Brushing hair sequence, 160. *See also* Task analysis

C

Chaining, 24–25, 146, 148–152, **199**
Challenging or problem behavior. *See also* Behaviors
  child's struggles with tasks in the sequence, 140, 144–145
  consequences of, 95–100
  extinction burst and, 93–94
  function of behaviors and, 86–95
  overview, 24, 85–86
Child behavior safety assessment, 47–48. *See also* Assessment
Choice, 17, 30
Classifying Stressors worksheet, 71, 72, 73, 76, 78, 80
Closed-ended activity
  definition of, **199**
  engagement in nonpreferred activities and, 52–53
  engagement in preferred activities and, 51–52
College goals, 2. *See also* Inclusive higher education programs
Communication
  emotional control of parents and, 94–95
  saying what you mean and, 91
  shared communication with professionals and, 3
Communication skills instruction, 25, 45
Community support, 71. *See also* Support networks
Consequences. *See also* Punishment; Reinforcement
  avoiding prompt dependency, 173–174
  child's struggles with tasks in the sequence, 139–140, 145
  definition of, **199**
  in the real world, 97–98

Consistency
  assessing, 72, 73, 77
  emotional control of parents and, 95
  extinction burst and, 93–94
  function of behaviors and, 90–91
  meaning what you say and, 91–92
  overview, 27, 31
  readiness of parents, 64, 65, 67, 79
Contrived reinforcement, 97, **199–200**. *See also* Reinforcement
Coping strategies, 67, 90, 95
Culture of dependence, xi–xii, 2

D

Daily living routines. *See also* Independent living skills; Routines; Task analysis
  breaking down for task analysis, 26–27
  following directions in context, 53–54
  giving directions and, 30–31
  modification and, 179–182
  overhelping and, 105–106
  picking the correct routine to start task analysis with, 154–157
  preparation and, 92–93
  reflecting on, 20–22
  reminders and directions and, 9–10
  responsibility for, 3
  from a single activity to a multistep process, 130–133
  verbal prompts and, 112–113
Data tracking
  readiness of parents, 66
  responsibilities of families in task analysis and, 28–30
Delay of rewards, 99–100
Dependence, culture of, xi–xii, 2
Destruction of property, 44–45, 47–48. *See also* Unsafe behaviors
Developmental disability (DD). *See* Intellectual or developmental disability (IDD)
Directions. *See also* Redirection
  ability to accept redirection, 55
  child's struggles with tasks in the sequence, 145
  daily living routines and, 9–10
  following directions in context, 53–54, 58–59
  following through with by parents, 86

foundational learning skills assessment, 58–59
learning to follow, 49–51
meaning what you say and, 91–92
responsibilities of families in task analysis and, 30–31
saying what you mean and, 91
Discrete trial teaching, 48–49
Distraction
child's struggles with tasks in the sequence, 137, 139
struggles with task analysis and, 148, 153
Dressing sequences, 159. *See also* Task analysis
Dysregulation. *See* Self-regulation; Unsafe behaviors

E

Education programs, 49–50. *See also* Inclusive higher education programs; School setting; Transition services
Electronic prompts, 9–10, 172. *See also* Prompting
Elopement, 42–43, 47–48, **200**
Emotion regulation. *See* Self-regulation
Emotional factors
assessing, 72, 73, 77
readiness of parents, 64, 67–68, 79, 94–95
Employment, 2, 17–19, 50
Engagement
"first, then" concept and, 57–58
in nonpreferred activities, 52–53
in preferred activities, 51–52
reinforcement and, 95–96
Environment. *See also* Supportive environment
child's struggles with tasks in the sequence, 139, 141, 143, 144
engagement in preferred activities and, 52
readiness of parents, 64, 68–69
safe environment, 39, 43
struggles with task analysis and, 148, 153
supporting independence and, 172–173
Escape functions of a behavior, 86, 88, 90, 139. *See also* Function of behaviors
"Everybody EATS," 87–90. *See also* Attention functions of a behavior; Escape functions of a behavior; Sensory (automatically) mediated behavior; Tangible functions of a behavior

Evidence-based practices
communication and social skills development and, 25
discrete trial teaching, 48–49
overview, 26, 197
task analysis and, 2–3, 24
External events
child's struggles with tasks in the sequence, 137, 139
struggles with task analysis and, 148, 153
Extinction burst, 93–94

F

Fading of prompts. *See also* Prompting
avoiding prompt dependency, 173–174
backward chaining and, 148
forward chaining and, 146, 148
methods of, 170–173
overview, 24–25, 106, 164–170
struggles with task analysis and, 154
targeting prompts to fade, 174–175
task analysis and, 145
time delay, 170–171
Financial independence, 20
"First, then" concept, 57–59
Following directions. *See* Directions
Following through
meaning what you say and, 91–92
overview, 86
saying what you mean and, 91
Food shopping sequence, 130–132. *See also* Task analysis
Forward chaining, 146, 148, **200**. *See also* Chaining
Foundational skills
ability to accept prompts, 54–55
ability to accept redirection, 55
engagement in nonpreferred activities, 52–53
engagement in preferred activities, 51–52
"first, then" concept, 57–58
following directions, 49–51, 53–54
overview, 37, 48–58
readiness assessment and, 59–60
repetitive and restrictive behaviors, 56–57
skills instruction and, 20
stereotypic behavior and, 55–56
Friend networks, 15–16. *See also* Support networks

Full model prompt (FMP), 108–109. *See also* Prompting
Full physical (FP) prompt. *See also* Prompting
    identifying the prompts activity and, 114–125
    overview, 107–108
    prompt fading and, 165–169
    task analysis and, 136
Function of behaviors. *See also* Behaviors; Challenging or problem behavior
    consistency and, 90–91
    "Everybody EATS," 87–90
    making a list of reinforcers and, 100
    making reinforcement more effective and, 98–102
    meaning what you say and, 91–92
    overview, 86–95
    preparation and, 92–93
    saying what you mean and, 91

G

Gestural prompts. *See also* Prompting
    identifying the prompts activity and, 114–125
    overview, 110
    prompt fading and, 165–169
    task analysis and, 136
Goals
    accommodation and, 182–186
    data tracking and, 29
    difference between modifications and prompts, 181–182
    for the future, 2
    modification and, 179–182, 183–186
    overview, 180–182

H

Hand-over-hand (HOH) prompt, 107–108, 136. *See also* Prompting
Helping children
    overhelping and, 105–106
    prompting and, 105–106
    task analysis and, 141–144
Higher education programs. *See* Inclusive higher education programs
Home environment, 68–69. *See also* Environment
Home living skills sequences, 160. *See also* Task analysis
Hygiene sequences, 159, 160. *See also* Task analysis

I

IEP meetings, 29
Inability to self-regulate, 45–48. *See also* Self-regulation; Unsafe behaviors
Inclusive higher education programs, 2, 13–15, 50. *See also* Services and service providers after graduation
Inclusive postsecondary education, 2, 13–15, 50. *See also* Transition services
Independence. *See also* Independent living skills
    desire for, 104–105
    modifications and accommodations and, 181–182, 186–185
    overview, xi–xiii, 197
    prompt fading and, 170–173
    task analysis and, 136, 145, 148, 153, 156
Independent living skills. *See also* Daily living routines; Independence
    data tracking and, 28–30
    learning to follow directions and, 50
    overview, 19–20
    prompting and, 105–106
    readiness assessment and, 59–60
    reflecting on, 20–22
Individuals with Disabilities Education Act (IDEA), 14, **200**
Intellectual disability (ID)
    definition of, **200**
    employment and, 17–19
    overview, 12
    social networks and friendships and, 15–16
Intellectual or developmental disability (IDD), xi, **200**. *See also* Intellectual disability (ID)
Internal events
    child's struggles with tasks in the sequence, 139
    struggles with task analysis and, 148, 153
Intrusive prompts, 108, 165. *See also* Prompting
Isolated skills, 162–163

L

Licensed behavior analyst (LBA), 12–13, **200**
Life events
    assessing, 72
    readiness of parents, 63, 65, 79
Listening, 86
Logistics
    assessing, 72
    readiness of parents, 63–64, 65–66, 68–69, 79

M

Making a bowl of cereal sequence, 161. *See also* Task analysis
Making lunch for school sequence, 158–159. *See also* Task analysis
Medical reasons for behavior
    pica (eating nonfood items) and, 44
    readiness assessment and, 37
Model prompts. *See also* Prompting
    identifying the prompts activity and, 114–125
    overview, 108–109
    prompt fading and, 165–169
    task analysis and, 136
Modifications. *See also* Accommodation; Goals
    accommodation over, 186–187
    definition of, **200**
    difference between modifications and prompts, 181–182
    overview, 179–182, 183–186
Morning routine sequence, 162–163. *See also* Task analysis
Most-to-least prompt hierarchy. *See also* Prompting
    gestural prompts and, 110
    model prompts and, 108–109
    overview, 107
    physical prompts and, 107–108
    positional prompts and, 110–111
    visual prompts and, 111–112
Motivation
    function of behaviors and, 86–95
    making reinforcement more effective and, 98–102
    overview, 86
    responsibilities of families in task analysis and, 31–32
    struggles with task analysis and, 154
Motor planning
    child's struggles with tasks in the sequence, 139, 142
    modifications and accommodations and, 184–185
    struggles with task analysis and, 153
Multistep routines, 129–133. *See also* Routines; Task analysis
Muscle weakness
    child's struggles with tasks in the sequence, 139
    struggles with task analysis and, 153

N

Natural reinforcement, 97, **200**. *See also* Reinforcement
Negative reinforcement, 96, **200**. *See also* Reinforcement
Nonfood items, eating, 44, 47–48. *See also* Unsafe behaviors
Nonpreferred activities, engagement in
    child's struggles with tasks in the sequence, 140
    "first, then" concept and, 57–58
    foundational learning skills assessment, 58–59
    overview, 52–53, 86

O

Obsessive-compulsive disorder (OCD), 56
Occupational therapists
    data tracking and, 29
    struggles with task analysis and, 153
OCD-like behaviors, 56. *See also* Repetitive behaviors; Restrictive behaviors
Online supports, 41. *See also* Support networks
Open-ended activity
    definition of, **200**
    engagement in nonpreferred activities and, 52–53
    engagement in preferred activities and, 51–52
Overhelping, 105–106

P

Packing a lunch sequence, 158–159. *See also* Task analysis
Parenting, 1–2, 94–95. *See also* Readiness of parents
Partial model prompt (PMP), 108–109. *See also* Prompting
Partial physical (PP) prompt. *See also* Prompting
  identifying the prompts activity and, 114–125
  overview, 107–108
  prompt fading and, 165–169
  task analysis and, 136
Physical aggression, 41–42, 47–48. *See also* Behaviors; Unsafe behaviors
Physical prompts. *See also* Prompting
  ability to accept prompts, 54–55
  forward chaining and, 146, 148
  identifying the prompts activity and, 114–125
  overview, 106–108
  prompt fading and, 165–169, 174–175
  task analysis and, 136
Physical therapists
  data tracking and, 29
  struggles with task analysis and, 153
Pica (eating nonfood items), 44, 47–48. *See also* Unsafe behaviors
Play routines, 57. *See also* Routines
Positional prompts. *See also* Prompting
  identifying the prompts activity and, 114–125
  overview, 110–111
  prompt fading and, 165–169
  task analysis and, 136
Positive reinforcement, 31, 96, **200**. *See also* Reinforcement
Postsecondary education. *See* Inclusive postsecondary education
Praise, 24, 31, 99. *See also* Positive reinforcement
Preferred activities, engagement in. *See also* Foundational skills
  child's struggles with tasks in the sequence, 140
  "first, then" concept and, 57–58
  foundational learning skills assessment, 58–59
  overview, 51–52, 86
Prerequisite skills, 16, 48, **200**. *See also* Foundational skills

Presentation accommodation, 183. *See also* Accommodation
Privacy, 104–105
Probe, 136, 148, **200**
Problem behavior. *See* Challenging or problem behavior
Prompt dependency, 106, 165, 173–174, **201**. *See also* Prompting
Prompting. *See also* Fading of prompts
  ability to accept, 54–55
  backward chaining and, 148
  difference between modifications and prompts, 181–182
  extinction burst and, 94
  forward chaining and, 146, 148
  foundational learning skills assessment, 58–59
  identifying the prompts activity, 114–125
  intrusive prompts and, 108
  modifications and accommodations and, 186–194
  overview, 24–25, 105–106
  prompting hierarchy, 146, 148, 166
  task analysis and, 136–137
  types of prompts, 106–113
Prompting hierarchy. *See also* Prompting
  forward chaining and, 146, 148
  prompt fading and, 166
Property destruction, 44–45, 47–48. *See also* Unsafe behaviors
Punishment. *See also* Consequences
  compared to reinforcement, 96–97
  definition of, **201**
  function of behaviors and, 88–90
  in the real world, 97–98

R

Readiness assessment. *See also* Assessment; Readiness of parents
  child behavior safety assessment, 47–48
  foundational learning skills assessment, 58–59
  foundational skills, 48–59
  overview, 3, 27, 36–37, 59–60
  unsafe behaviors and, 37–48
Readiness of parents. *See also* Parenting; Readiness assessment
  assessing, 63–75, 102–103
  extinction burst and, 93–94

overview, 62–63, 74–81
preparation and, 92–93
self-regulation and, 94–95
Recording routines. *See also* Routines
data tracking and, 29–30
prompt fading and, 166
readiness of parents, 66
task analysis and, 134
Redirection. *See also* Directions
ability to accept, 55
definition of, **201**
following through with, 86
foundational learning skills assessment, 58–59
repetitive and restrictive behaviors, 56–57
stereotypic behavior and, 55–56
Reinforcement. *See also* Consequences; Reinforcers
avoiding prompt dependency, 173–174
child's struggles with tasks in the sequence, 139–140
compared to punishment, 96–97
consistency and, 90–91
contrived reinforcement, 97, **199–200**
definition of, **201**
function of behaviors and, 87–90
making more effective, 98–102
modifications and accommodations and, 186–194
natural reinforcement, 97, **200**
negative reinforcement, 96, **200**
overview, 95–100
positive reinforcement, 31, 96
property destruction and, 45
in the real world, 97–98
responsibilities of families in task analysis and, 31–32
struggles with task analysis and, 154
Reinforcers. *See also* Reinforcement
child's struggles with tasks in the sequence, 140
making a list of, 100
making reinforcement more effective and, 98–102
struggles with task analysis and, 148, 154
Reminders, 9–10, 172
Repetitive behaviors, 56–57. *See also* Behaviors
Replacement behaviors, 45. *See also* Behaviors
Response accommodation, 183. *See also* Accommodation
Restrictive behaviors, 56–57. *See also* Behaviors

Rewards, 24, 38, 46, 96. *See also* Positive reinforcement; Reinforcement
Routines. *See also* Daily living routines; Task analysis
data tracking and, 28–30
following directions in context, 53–54
multistep routines, 129–133
overview, 25
ownership of, xii
picking the correct routine to start task analysis with, 154–157
preparation and, 92–93
readiness of parents, 65, 66
repetitive and restrictive behaviors, 56–57
situational routines, 140, 141, 144
struggles with task analysis and, 153
unsafe behaviors and, 38
verbal prompts and, 112–113

S

Safe environment, 39, 43. *See also* Environment; Unsafe behaviors
Safety skills. *See also* Unsafe behaviors
elopement and, 43
overview, 38–39
readiness assessment and, 59–60
School setting, 29, 49–50, 186
Section 504 of the Rehabilitation Act of 1973, 14, **201**
Self-control, 51–53. *See also* Self-regulation
Self-direction, 50–51
Self-injurious behavior. *See also* Unsafe behaviors
child behavior safety assessment, 47–48
overview, 39–41
stereotypic behavior and, 56
Self-regulation
child behavior safety assessment, 47–48
definition of, **201**
inability to self-regulate, 45–47
readiness of parents, 69, 94–95
Sensory (automatically) mediated behavior. *See also* Behaviors; Function of behaviors; Self-injurious behavior; Stereotypic behavior; Unsafe behaviors
definition of, **201**
elopement, 42–43
modifications and accommodations and, 185–186

Sensory (automatically) mediated behavior (*continued*)
  overview, 39, 86, 89–90, 100
  self-injurious behavior, 39–41
Services and service providers after graduation. *See also* Inclusive postsecondary education; Transition services
  data tracking and, 29
  lack of, 12–13
Setting accommodation, 183. *See also* Accommodation
Setting the table sequence, 162. *See also* Task analysis
Showering sequence, 157–158. *See also* Task analysis
Situational routines, 140, 141, 144. *See also* Routines
Skills instruction. *See* Foundational skills
Social connections, 15–16. *See also* Support networks
Social skills instruction, 16, 25
Socially mediated behavior. *See also* Behaviors; Self-injurious behavior; Unsafe behaviors
  definition of, **201**
  elopement, 42–43
  overview, 39
  self-injurious behavior, 39–41
Solutions, brainstorming, 71, 73, 76, 77, 78, 81
Special education programs, 48–49
Staying on task. *See also* Foundational skills
  ability to accept redirection, 55
  "first, then" concept and, 57–58
  nonpreferred activities and, 52–53
  preferred activities and, 51–52
  repetitive and restrictive behaviors, 56–57
  stereotypic behavior and, 55–56
Stereotypic behavior, 52, 55–56, **201**. *See also* Sensory (automatically) mediated behavior
Stressors
  assessing for, 71, 72–73, 80
  readiness of parents, 69
Structure, 30–31
Supervision, xi–xii
Support groups, 16
Support networks. *See also* Supportive environment
  assessing, 72, 73, 77
  readiness of parents, 64, 70–71, 79

Supportive environment. *See also* Environment; Support networks
  assessing, 72, 73, 77
  readiness of parents, 64, 68–69, 79
Systematic fading of prompts. *See* Fading of prompts; Prompting

T

Taking off shoes sequence, 161. *See also* Task analysis
Tangible functions of a behavior, 86, 89, 90, 100. *See also* Function of behaviors
Task analysis. *See also* Daily living routines; Multistep routines; Routines
  child's struggles with tasks in the sequence, 137, 139–146
  definition of, **201**
  engagement in nonpreferred activities and, 52
  food shopping sequence, 130–132
  forward and backward chaining and, 146, 148–152
  how routines are broken down for, 26–27
  overview, 2–3, 12, 24–25, 129–130
  picking the correct routine to start with, 154–157
  prompting and, 165–166
  responsibilities of families in, 27–32
  sequences for other everyday tasks, 157–163
  simple task analysis, 133–151
  from a single activity to a multistep process, 130–133
  stringing together isolated skills to create a sequence and, 162–163
  struggles with, 148, 153
  toothbrushing sequence, 132–137, 138
  verbal prompts and, 112–113
  what tasks should be broken down for, 26
Task Analysis Data Worksheet, 134, 135, 137, 138, 142, 143, 146, 148–152
Technology in prompting, 9–10, 172
Telehealth services, 41
Time commitment
  assessing, 72, 77
  readiness of parents, 64, 66, 79
Time delay, 170–171, 174–175. *See also* Fading of prompts
Time management accommodation, 183. *See also* Accommodation

Timers, 9–10, 172
Toothbrushing sequence. *See also* Task analysis
  child's struggles with tasks in the sequence, 142, 143, 144–145
  forward and backward chaining and, 146, 148–152
  overview, 132–137, 138
  struggles with, 148, 153
Total task chaining, 146. *See also* Chaining
Tracking data, 28–30
Transition services, 12–15, 16–17, 19–20. *See also* Inclusive postsecondary education; Services and service providers after graduation
Troubleshooting Worksheet, 146, 147

U

Unsafe behaviors. *See also* Behaviors
  aggressive behaviors, 41–42, 47–48
  child behavior safety assessment, 47–48
  elopement, 42–43
  inability to self-regulate, 45–47
  overview, 37–47
  pica (eating nonfood items) and, 44, 47–48
  property destruction, 44–45, 47–48
  readiness assessment and, 59–60
  self-injurious behavior, 39–41, 47–48, 56
  stereotypic behavior, 52, 55–56

V

Verbal aggression. *See* Aggressive behaviors
Verbal praise. *See* Positive reinforcement; Praise; Reinforcement
Verbal program, 112–113
Verbal prompts. *See also* Prompting
  identifying the prompts activity and, 114–125
  overview, 112–113
  prompt fading and, 165–169

Video prompts, 171–172. *See also* Prompting
Video recording of routines. *See also* Routines
  data tracking and, 29–30
  prompt fading and, 166
  readiness of parents, 66
  task analysis and, 134
Visual prompts. *See also* Prompting
  overview, 54–55, 108, 111–112
  prompt fading and, 171–172
  task analysis and, 136
  visual schedule, 148
Vocational rehabilitation programming, 14–15. *See also* Services and service providers after graduation

W

Washing hair sequence, 158. *See also* Task analysis
Washing hands sequence, 160. *See also* Task analysis
Workforce rehabilitation programming, 14–15. *See also* Services and service providers after graduation
Worksheets
  Assessing for Barriers worksheet, 71, 76, 78, 79
  Brainstorming Solutions worksheet, 71, 76, 77, 78, 81
  Classifying Stressors worksheet, 71, 72, 73, 76, 78, 80
  Task Analysis Data Worksheet, 134, 135, 137, 138, 142, 143, 146, 148–152
  Troubleshooting Worksheet, 146, 147
Written prompts, 171–172. *See also* Prompting

Z

Zipping jacket sequence, 161. *See also* Task analysis

About the Authors

Kristin Lombardi, MA, BCBA, helps children and families prepare for independent living in her private practice in Locust Valley, New York. With a background in special education, psychology, and behavior analysis, she works with preschoolers through young adults with varying support needs.

Christine Drew, PhD, BCBA-D, is Assistant Professor of Special Education at Auburn University, where she teaches graduate and undergraduate courses and works with Auburn's inclusive higher education program for students with intellectual disabilities. Prior to becoming a professor, she ran a middle school behavior program.